SELF-ASSESSMENT PICTURE TESTS IN VETERINARY MEDICINE

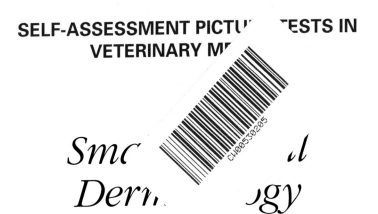

Small Animal Dermatology

Edited by
Barbara A Kummel DVM
Veterinary Referral Associates, Inc.
Maryland, U.S.A.

⋈ Wolfe

Copyright © 1994 Times Mirror International Publishers Limited
Published in 1994 by Mosby–Wolfe Publishing, an imprint of Times Mirror
International Publishers Limited
Printed by Grafos, S. A. Arte sobre papel
ISBN 0 7234 1944 2

For full details of all Times Mirror International Publishers Limited titles please
write to Times Mirror International Publishers Limited, Lynton House, 7–12
Tavistock Square, London WC1H 9LB, England.

A CIP catalogue record for this book is available from the British Library.

Library of Congress Cataloging-in-Publication Data has been applied for.

NAMES AND ADDRESSES
OF CONTRIBUTORS

Dr Barbara A. Kummel, Veterinary Referral Associates, Inc., 15021 Dufief Mill Road, Gaithersburg, Maryland 20878, U.S.A.

With additional contributions by

Dr Stephen D. White, Department of Clinical Studies, Colorado State University, College of Veterinary Medicine and Biomedical Sciences, Fort Collins, Colorado, U.S.A.

Dr Michael H. Goldschmidt, Laboratory of Pathology, University of Pennsylvania, School of Veterinary Medicine, Philadelphia, Pennsylvania, U.S.A.

Dr Diane E. Bevier, North Carolina State University – S.V.M., Raleigh, North Carolina, U.S.A.

Dr Karen A. Moriello, University of Wisconsin, Madison, Wisconsin, U.S.A.

1 Head and neck excoriations are very common presenting clinical signs in feline dermatology. This middle-aged female feline patient presented with a history of warm weather facial pruritus, resulting in excoriations, which had become progressively more severe each year.
(a) What is the diagnosis?
(b) How would you treat this patient?
(c) What are other causes of head and/or neck excoriations in the feline patient?

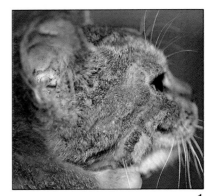
1

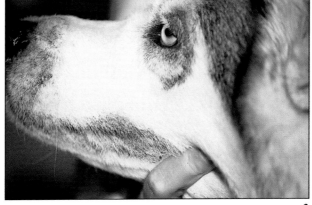
2

2 This 2-year-old female Siberian husky has a 6-month history of non-pruritic encrusted lesions bilaterally around the periocular areas and the commissures of the lips. The dog is being fed a well-balanced, commercially available diet.
(a) What are your differential diagnoses?
(b) What one diagnostic test would be most indicated?

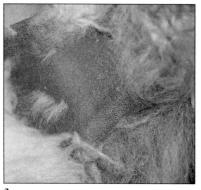

3

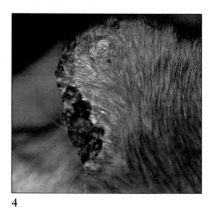

4

3 This 18-month-old male intact Keeshond has a 2-month history of progressive hair loss and hyperpigmentation involving the entire circumference of the neck, the areas caudal to the scapulas and the tail. Thyroid testing, as well as a complete blood count and chemistry profile, are within normal limits. The patient is non-pruritic. The truncal hair coat has developed a fine, cottony, 'puppy-like' texture. The testes palpate normally and there are no signs of feminisation. A biopsy of the skin reveals 'hair cycle growth arrest with occasional follicular atrophy, suggestive of an endocrinopathy'.
(a) What is your most likely diagnosis?
(b) How would you confirm your diagnosis?

4 The ear pinnae of a 9-year-old female spayed mixed-breed dog is pictured. This patient has cold agglutinin disease, a rare (controversial) skin disease of the dog and cat. It is an autoimmune disease associated with low temperature reacting IgM autoantibodies (0 – 30° C).
(a) List three differential diagnoses.
(b) List two appropriate diagnostic tests.

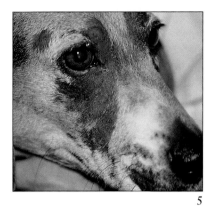

5

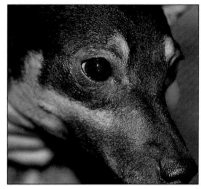

6

5 This 8-year-old Beagle presented with a several-month history of gradual facial hair loss. The patient was non-pruritic. Skin scrapings and fungal cultures were negative. Histopathologic examination showed a normal epidermis and atrophic hair follicles. The follicular bulbs were surrounded by a mixed mononuclear infiltrate.
(a) What is the diagnosis of this very rare disease of the dog and cat?
(b) What is the treatment?
(c) What is the prognosis?

6 This 5-year-old mixed-breed dog has a 2-year history of pruritic dermatitis involving the periocular areas and muzzle. The ears, axillary areas and feet are also quite pruritic. The intensity of the pruritus is more severe during times of high tree and weed pollen count. The pruritus is alleviated by anti-inflammatory doses of corticosteroids.
(a) What is the most likely diagnosis?
(b) Which breeds of dogs are known to have a predilection for this hereditary disease?
(c) What is the average age of onset of clinical signs?
(d) Is there any known sex predilection?
(e) Which antibody or antibodies are thought to mediate the disease?

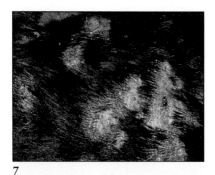

7

7 This 6-month-old mixed-breed puppy is presented with a 1-month history of pruritic multi-focal areas of hair loss on the trunk.
(a) List the most common differential diagnoses.
(b) What tests and/or procedures would you perform to confirm your diagnosis?

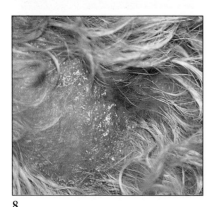

8

8 This area of acute moist dermatitis (hot spot) occurred in a 3-year-old Saint Bernard.
(a) What is (are) the most common age(s), breed(s) and sex(es) of dogs that present with this cutaneous sign?
(b) What types of underlying diseases are these lesions usually secondary to?
(c) How do you determine whether or not systemic antibiotics are necessary in the treatment of this disease?

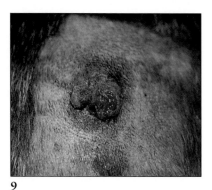

9

9 An apocrine adenoma on the mid-back of a 3-year-old Bull mastiff is shown.
(a) Is this a common tumour in the dog?
(b) Are the lesions usually solitary or multiple?
(c) What is the average size of the tumour?
(d) Is this 3-year-old patient the 'classic' age for the development of this tumour?

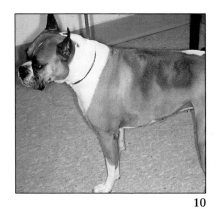

10

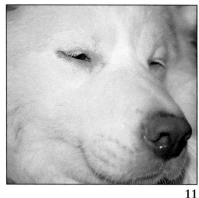

11

10 The hyperpigmented/alopecic areas on this 5-year-old spayed female Boxer have been present for 3 months, but have previously occurred and resolved in past years. No pruritus, or any other clinical signs, are noted by the owner. Skin scrapings, fungal culture, haemogram, serum chemistry panel, adrenal and thyroid function tests are all negative or normal.
(a)   What is your tentative diagnosis?
(b)   How could you confirm this?

11 This 6-year-old female spayed Samoyed presented with decreased pigment involving the planum nasale, lips and periocular areas. Physical examination also revealed photophobia and uveitis. This patient has Vogt–Koyanagi–Harada-like syndrome.
(a)   Is there any recognised breed predilection in the dog?
(b)   Has this disease been recognised in the cat?
(c)   What are the two major cutaneous changes?
(d)   Which is more important to the health of the patient, the cutaneous changes or the uveitis?

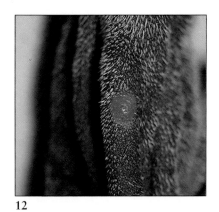

12

12 This young Chinese Shar pei presented with a 1 cm alopecic, erythematous mass on the hindleg. Histopathologic examination revealed a fibrous histiocytoma.
(a) What is the average age that canine patients are presented with these tumours?
(b) Are the tumours solitary or multiple?
(c) What are the most common sites of these tumours?

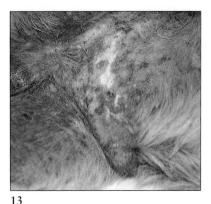

13

13 This patient developed severe, generalised, very painful ulcerations several days after initiating a course of antibiotics prescribed for dog fight lacerations.
(a) What are your differential diagnoses?
(b) What is the diagnosis?
(c) What are the two major groups of drugs responsible for initiating this potentially fatal disease in the dog?
(d) Is this disease common, uncommon or rare?

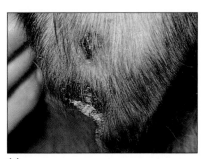

14

14 This 12-year-old mixed-breed dog presented with necrosis of the ear pinnal tips, tail tip and footpads. Involved areas were painful, but otherwise the patient was asymptomatic.
(a) What are your differential diagnoses?
(b) What is/are your most important diagnostic test(s)?

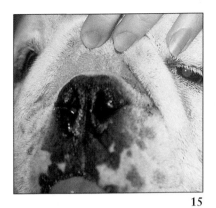

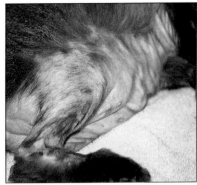

15

16

15 This area of facial fold
dermatitis is seen in a young male
intact English bulldog. The patient's
face is moderately pruritic, and the
owner complains of an 'odour'
noticed about the face and head.
(a) What other types of fold
dermatitis are recognised in the
dog?
(b) What are the typical breed, age,
sex or other factors causing an
increased risk for fold dermatitis?
(c) What is the treatment?

16 The middle-aged female spayed
cat shown has a seasonal condition
with pruritus which causes licking
and partial alopecia involving the
lateral thoracic areas, abdomen and
rear legs. The tentative diagnosis is
feline allergic inhalant disease
(atopy).
(a) What other skin changes have
been reported in feline patients with
allergic inhalant disease (atopy)?
(b) Is there a known age, breed or
sex predilection for this
(hereditary?) allergic disease in the
feline?
(c) Has IgE been identified in the
cat?

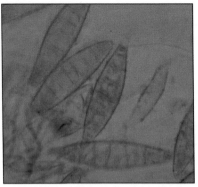

17

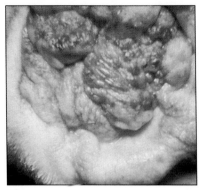

18

17 A 6-month-old female Siamese kitten is presented to you by the owner with the complaint of pruritus, generalised areas of hair loss and excessive scaling. Examination of the kitten reveals multifocal areas with broken stubbly hairs, excessive scaling and erythematous borders. Skin scrapings and Wood's lamp examination of new lesions also are negative. A toothbrush fungal culture, however, shows growth on dermatophyte Test Media at 10 days. The gross colony is white and fluffy with sporulation of the organism (pictured).
(a) What is your diagnosis?
(b) What are your treatment goals?

18 An 11-year-old neutered male domestic short-haired cat presents with a history of a chronic infection of the external ear canal. Examination of the ear reveals multiple 1–2 mm, slightly raised, brownish-black, intra-epidermal protuberances.
(a) What is your diagnosis?
(b) What is the most likely cause of these lesions?

19 This 7-year-old male intact Wire Haired Fox terrier has a 4-month history of alopecia and hyperpigmentation involving a 2 cm area of the dorsal tail, approximately 5 cm from the base of the tail. The affected area palpates thicker than normal-appearing, neighbouring skin. Neither pruritus nor pain has been noticed by the owner. Skin scrapings and fungal culture are negative. The testes palpate normally.

(a) What is your tentative diagnosis?

(b) How would you confirm this diagnosis?

(c) What is the treatment?

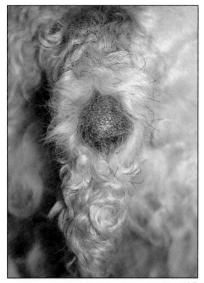

19

20 The ventral neck of a 5-year-old female spayed Shih tzu is shown. The skin condition is described as being seborrhoea oleosa. The patient is quite pruritic in involved areas and is responsive to combinations of corticosteroids, antibiotics and anti-yeast medications.

(a) Is seborrhoea oleosa usually a primary or a secondary cutaneous change?

(b) What are the most common causes of secondary seborrhoea oleosa?

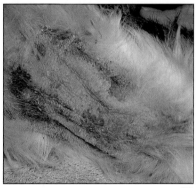

20

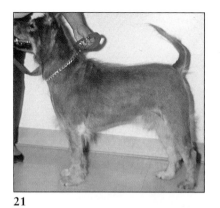

21

21 This 2-year-old male Chow Chow has a 1-year history of severe truncal alopecia with moderate scaling. There is no pruritus as reported by the owner. Skin scrapings, fungal culture, haemogram and serum chemistry panel are all negative or normal.
(a) What is your tentative diagnosis?
(b) How would you confirm this?
(c) What is the treatment?

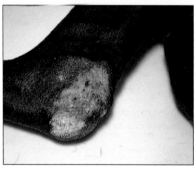

22

22 The left hock of a 13-year-old Chocolate Labrador retriever is shown. There is alopecia, inflammation and some secondary bacterial infection.
(a) What is the diagnosis?
(b) What are some complicating factors?

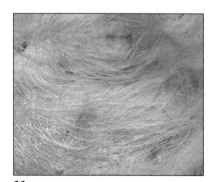

23

23 The erythematous, scaling lesions on the abdomen and prepuce of a 14-year-old West Highland White terrier are shown. Erythematous ulcerative lesions were present at numerous mucocutaneous junctions. A histopathologic diagnosis of cutaneous lymphosarcoma was made on multiple biopsies taken from affected areas.
(a) Name the clinically defined stages of this tumour as found most frequently in the dog.
(b) Which stage is depicted?

24 This 1-year-old spayed female Irish terrier has a 5-month history of generalised nonpruritic alopecia . The dog was spayed at 5.5 months of age. The patient had been given an adequate dosage of thyroid supplementation, on an empirical basis, for 2 months, without results. Skin biopsy reveals 'hair growth cycle arrest with occasional follicular atrophy, suggestive of an endocrinopathy'.

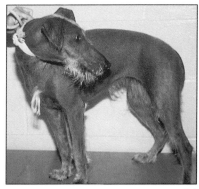

24

(a) What is your tentative diagnosis?

(b) How would this be confirmed?

25 This 3-year-old indoor/outdoor cat developed these non-healing areas of soft-tissue abscessation with ulcers and draining fistulas. Direct smears of the discharge revealed acid-fast organisms.

(a) What is the most likely diagnosis and organism(s) responsible for this disease?

(b) What area(s) of the cat's body is/are most frequently involved and why?

(c) How might you manage this case?

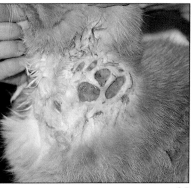

25

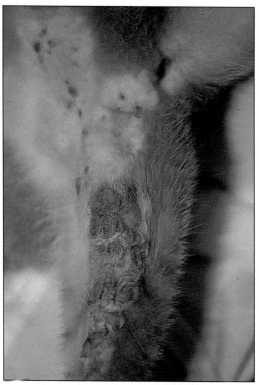

26

26 This 3-year-old domestic short-haired cat has an erythematous, ulcerated lesion on the caudal aspect of the right rear leg. The owners report that the lesion has been present for 18 months. They also report that the cat grooms (licks) the area excessively, especially during the autumn months of high weed pollen count and high mould count. Histopathologic examination of a biopsy taken revealed a hyperplastic, superficial and deep perivascular dermatitis with eosinophils. Blood eosinophilia was also present.
(a) What is the most likely diagnosis?
(b) What other differential diagnoses would you consider?
(c) In addition to the caudal thigh, what other area of the cat is most predisposed to the development of these lesions?

27 A young female spayed Chow Chow is presented with mucocutaneous ulceration of several weeks' duration. The patient is not pruritic and appears to be painful.
(a) List five differential diagnoses.
(b) How would you make a definitive diagnosis?
(c) What does cytologic examination of the exudate from the surface of the lesions reveal?
(d) What is your treatment protocol?

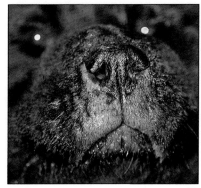

27

28 This 9-year-old female spayed domestic short-haired white cat has a 2-year history of poorly controlled diabetes mellitus. She presented with large areas of epidermal sloughing, mainly involving her trunk. The skin peeled off easily when scraped or combed. The patient was anorectic and lethargic.
(a) What is the most probable cause of the skin lesions (and of the diabetes mellitus)?
(b) How would you confirm your diagnosis(es)?
(c) What is the prognosis?

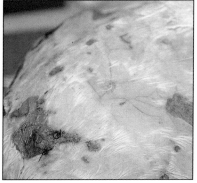

28

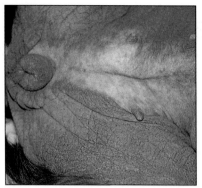

29

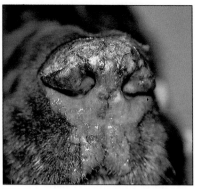

30

29 This 7-year-old black female intact American Cocker spaniel has a 5-month history of alopecia, hyperpigmentation, and moderate pruritus involving the perineal area, abdomen and medial thighs. Physical examination reveals hypertrophy and hyperpigmentation of the perianal and vulvar skin. Skin scrapings, a fungal culture, complete blood count and chemistry profile were within 'normal' limits. Biopsies of the involved skin revealed acanthosis, hyperpigmentation and hair growth cycle arrest. This is suggestive of an endocrine imbalance. No other clinical signs were present.
(a) What is your tentative diagnosis?
(b) How would you confirm your diagnosis?

30 The ulcerated nose of a female spayed mixed-breed black Labrador retriever is pictured. The condition has been present for greater than 6 months, and has become progressively more severe. The diagnosis is discoid lupus erythematous.
(a) This disease is considered to be a benign variant of which other canine autoimmune skin disorder?
(b) Is discoid lupus erythematous (DLE) always an 'easy' disease to treat?

31 This 7-year-old domestic medium-haired white cat presented with hair loss around the neck of several months' duration. The patient was non-pruritic. A complete blood count and chemistry profile were within normal limits, and the cat had not received any medication for almost a year. A resting free T4 and total T4 were very low.

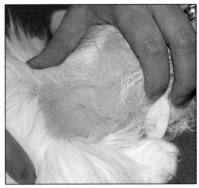

31

(a) What is the diagnosis?
(b) How common is this disease in the feline?
(c) What is the treatment?

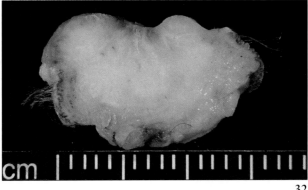

32

32 A 3-year-old Beagle on a drug study at the 'XYZ' Pharmaceutical Company has a 2.5 cm diameter, ulcerated, endophytic mass surgically excised from the gluteal region. The cross section of this mass is pictured. On histopathologic examination, the mass was diagnosed as a squamous cell carcinoma. What is the likely etiology of this tumour?

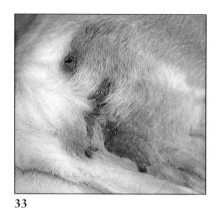

33

33 The 3-year-old mixed hound, pictured, is diabetic. Recently, she developed ulcerated nodules, abscesses and cellulitis involving the caudal thigh and left hind leg. Severe popliteal lymphadenopathy was present at the time of examination. Direct smear of some discharge from the lesions revealed organisms that were branched at right angles, beaded in some areas and partially acid-fast.
(a) What is the most likely diagnosis?
(b) How would you confirm this diagnosis?
(c) What therapy would be appropriate for this patient?

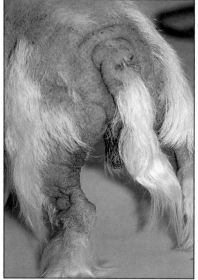

34

34 This 4-year-old West Highland White terrier presented with a pruritic, erythematous, papulocrustous dermatitis which was most severe over the rump, tail, head and caudal thighs. Fleas and flea excreta were found using a flea comb. An immediate (10-minute) intradermal skin test was negative for flea saliva.
(a) What is the most likely diagnosis?
(b) How do you explain the negative intradermal skin test reaction in light of the probable clinical diagnosis?
(c) What other differential diagnoses would you include?

35 A 6-year-old female spayed West Highland White terrier is presented with idiopathic seborrhoea (an inherited disorder of keratinisation). The owner complains that the patient becomes intensely pruritic if she is not bathed in an anti-seborrhoeic shampoo 2 – 3 times per week. The pruritus does not respond to antibiotics, anti-parasiticidals, antihistamines or other conventional therapy for pruritus. Close examination of the patient's skin reveals thick yellowish accumulations of debris. An impression smear is made of this debris, heat fixed and stained with a fast Giemsa stain. Microscopic examination reveals wax, occasional nucleated epithelial cells, rare neutrophils and at least ten *Malassezia* organisms per high power field. Cytologic examination of ear smears from the same patient reveal similar findings.

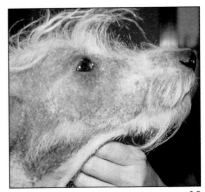

35

(a)   What is your diagnosis?
(b)   What role does the *Malassezia* play in this patient's skin disease?
(c)   What are possible therapies?

36 This young male intact red and rust Dobermann pinscher presented with a complaint of 'dandruff'.
(a)   What is the dermatologic name for this condition?
(b)   List five possible causes?

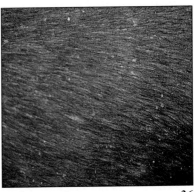

36

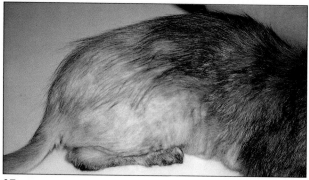

37

37 This 3-year-old female cat has self-induced hair loss involving the caudal half of her body, including her tail and rear legs. The diagnosis is flea bite hypersensitivity.
(a) How would you make this diagnosis?
(b) What are the differential diagnoses?
(c) What is the most common 'misdiagnosis'?

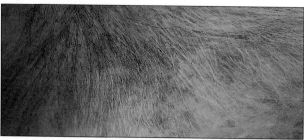

38

38 A 5-year-old mixed-breed dog presents with a 2-year history of non-seasonal pruritus and an erythematous papular eruption. The clinical diagnosis is food hypersensitivity.
(a) What is the 'classical' presentation of food hypersensitivity in the canine?
(b) How is the diagnosis of food hypersensitivity made?
(c) Are dogs with food hypersensitivity responsive to corticosteroids?

39 This 10-week-old Golden retriever puppy presented with a 2-week history of progressing truncal nodules. The lesions were painful and non-pruritic. The owner reported that the lesions would often open and drain a haemo-purulent, greasy material. Bacterial and fungal cultures of the exudate revealed no growth.
(a) What is the most likely diagnosis?
(b) What are the most important diagnostic tests?
(c) What is the treatment?

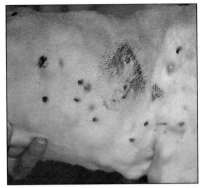

39

40 This 9-week-old male Akita puppy presented with a 10-day history of hair loss, swelling and pain involving the muzzle, periocular areas and ear pinnae. The submandibular lymph nodes were very enlarged.
(a) What is the diagnosis?
(b) What is the treatment?
(c) What is the pathogenesis?

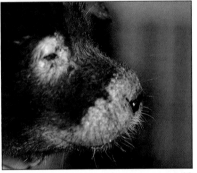

40

41 This 7-year-old female spayed mixed American Cocker spaniel presented with hyperkeratosis of all footpads. The condition was asymptomatic.
(a) What is this condition called?
(b) What are some underlying diseases which cause this condition?

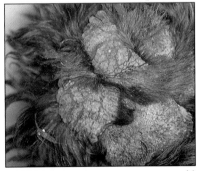

41

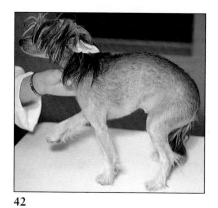

42 This 1-year-old female intact dog is presented for routine vaccination and examination. She has near total truncal hair loss, with long hair on her head, neck, distal legs and tail.
(a) Does this dog have a skin disease?
(b) What breed of dog is she?
(c) What are the two varieties of this breed?

42

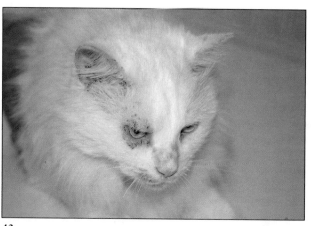

43

43 This 3-year-old male intact domestic medium-haired cat presented with alopecia, erythema and crusting involving the muzzle, bridge of nose, periocular area and ear pinnae. The patient is non-pruritic and has not responded to an appropriate course of antibiotics and insecticidal dips.
(a) What are your primary differential diagnoses?
(b) What is the most important diagnostic test?
(c) Are there any recognised age, breed or sex predilections in the feline?

44 This 3-year-old female spayed feline patient presented with a 2-year history of non-seasonal facial and neck pruritus which resulted in excoriations. The diagnosis is food hypersensitivity.

(a) How would you make this diagnosis?

(b) What are other causes of head and neck excoriations in the feline patient?

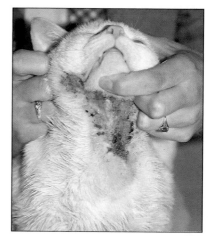

44

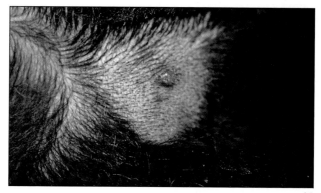

45

45 An erythematous, button-like mass on the rear leg of a 6-month-old black Scottish terrier is pictured. The area has been shaved for better visualisation. The lesion is non-pruritic and non-painful.

(a) What is your diagnosis?

(b) What is the biological behaviour of this lesion?

(c) Are there any dog breeds which are at greater risk than the average dog population for developing this lesion?

(d) At what age does this lesion most frequently develop?

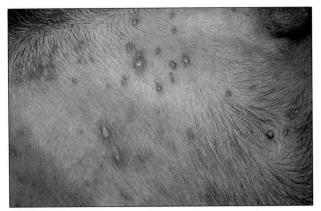

46

46 This 3-month-old red and rust Dobermann pinscher puppy is presented for a routine examination and vaccinations. Physical examination reveals a number of small, superficial pustules on the skin of the caudal abdomen. The lesions do not involve the hair follicles.
(a) What is the diagnosis?
(b) What is the underlying aetiology?
(c) What are your treatment options?

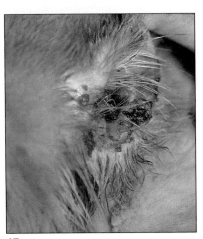

47

47 This 11-year-old male neutered Persian cat presented with a 5-month history of waxing and waning crusts, erosions and ulceration involving the nose, lips and ear pinnae and, to a lesser degree, the periocular areas. The patient was non-pruritic and apparently in pain.
(a) If the owner was unable to afford any diagnostic testing, how would you treat this cat? (The only other option is euthanasia.)
(b) Why did you choose this course of treatment?

48 The abdomen of an 11-year-old intact female mixed Miniature Poodle is pictured. The severely ulcerated lesions have been noticed by the owner for only about a week. The lesions are mildly pruritic and appear to be painful.

(a) What is your most probable diagnosis?

(b) How is your diagnosis made?

(c) Why is there a serous exudate on the skin surface?

(d) What is the biological behaviour of this tumour?

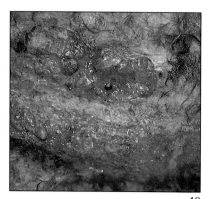

48

49 This 3-year-old fawn-coloured Great Dane presented with a 2-week history of lesions, which initially resembled small hives. The hairs appeared to stand on end and involved the skin over the back and sides. The lesions soon progressed to small patches of alopecia, giving the dog's coat a 'moth-eaten' appearance (**A**). On examination of the abdominal skin, circular areas of scaling with mildly erythematous cankers were found (**B**). The patient was mildly pruritic.

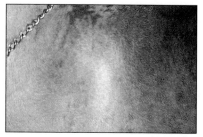

49A

(a) What is the most likely diagnosis?

(b) What are the lesions in **B** called?

What do these lesions represent?

(c) What therapy would you recommend for this patient?

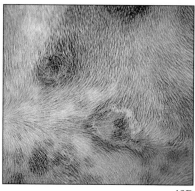

49B

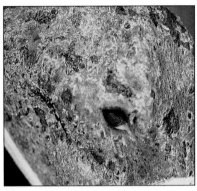

50

50 This 7-month-old male Dobermann pinscher presented with a several-month history of progressive, generalised alopecia and scaling. Histopathologic examination of skin biopsies revealed lamellar ichthyosis.
(a) How common is this disease in the dog?
(b) Is the Dobermann pinscher predisposed?
(c) What is the treatment?

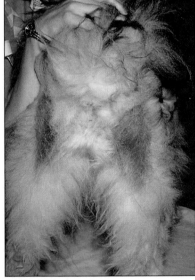

51

51 This 6-year-old spayed female Keeshond has a 1-year history of bilateral, hyperpigmented, non-pruritic alopecia involving the caudal thighs. Skin scrapings, fungal culture, complete blood count, chemistry profile, adrenal gland and thyroid function tests were all negative or within normal limits. A skin biopsy submitted for histopathologic examination revealed hair growth cycle arrest with occasional follicular atrophy, suggestive of an endocrine imbalance.
(a) What is your tentative diagnosis?
(b) How would you confirm your diagnosis?

52 This 5-year-old Old English sheepdog presented with rapid development of alopecic, erythematous, coalescing plaques involving the entire skin surface. The histopathologic diagnosis is malignant histiocytosis.
(a) What non-cutaneous signs often accompany this disease?
(b) Is there any breed predilection?
(c) What is the prognosis?

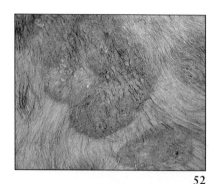

52

53 This young kitten is presented with the complaint of head shaking and scratching. Visual examination of the external ear canals reveals black debris.
(a) What is your most likely diagnosis?
(b) Can this diagnosis be confirmed?
(c) What is an appropriate therapy?

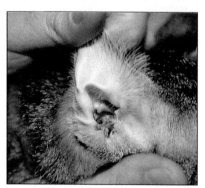

53

54 This 7-year-old male Great Dane has developed draining lesions involving the callous areas of both elbows.
(a) What is this disorder called?
(b) What is the underlying pathomechanism of this condition?
(c) What other areas of the body may be affected?
(d) What are the treatment recommendations?
(e) What is the long-term prognosis for this condition?

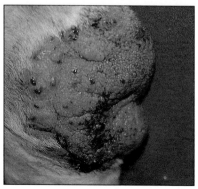

54

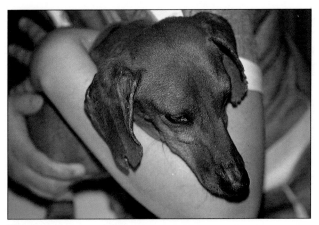

55

55 This 6-year-old miniature short-haired Dachshund has bilateral ear pinnal alopecia with scalloping (notching) of the ear pinnal margins. The patient is not pruritic and has no history of ear infections. Multiple skin scrapings were negative for mites.
(a) What is your tentative diagnosis?
(b) How would you confirm your diagnosis?
(c) What is the treatment?

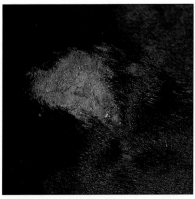

56

56 The 12-year-old male neutered Labrador retriever pictured has deep pyoderma/cellulitis over his hips. The condition has been present for several months and is painful and mildly pruritic.
(a) What structures of the skin are involved in this infection?
(b) What is (are) the most likely underlying disorders which can cause this condition?
(c) What systemic sequel may result from this type of infection?

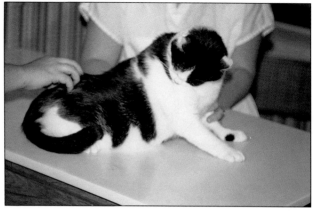

57

57 This 9-year-old domestic short-haired cat has a history of extreme irritability/sensitivity when stroked over the midlumbar back region. Stroking the cat in this area results in the cat biting the owner or himself, and a noticeable twitching or rippling of the muscles and skin in the area. The cat will occasionally turn and growl at the lumbar area and will spontaneously attack and chew the area.
(a)   What is the probable diagnosis?
(b)   What diagnostics are indicated in an attempt to find the cause of this disorder?

58 The cross-section of a mass that was removed from the elbow region of a 2-year-old Great Dane is pictured. The mass had been present for several weeks.
(a)   What is your diagnosis?
(b)   What is the prognosis?
(c)   At what other sites do these lesions occur in the dog?
(d)   What is another term used to describe these lesions?

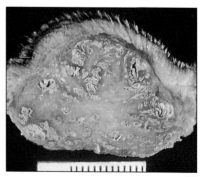

58

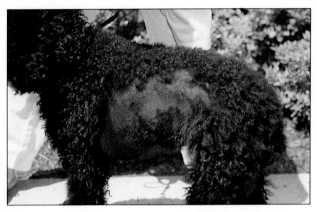

59

59 This 3-year-old female Portuguese water dog presented with a history of progressive truncal hair loss. The patient was non-pruritic and showed no signs of systemic disease. A thyroid profile, complete blood count and chemistry profile were normal.
(a) What disease does this patient have?
(b) List three major differential diagnoses.
(c) What is the treatment?
(d) Other than the Portuguese water dog, list several other breeds of dogs which appear to be predisposed to developing this condition.

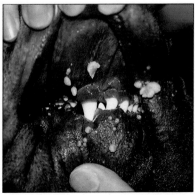

60

60 Lesions have rapidly developed on the lips and mouth of this 7-month-old male Chinese Shar pei .
(a) What is the diagnosis?
(b) What is the aetiology of these lesions?
(c) What is the most common site of the development of these lesions and what clinical signs may be associated with these lesions?
(d) Is there any breed predilection for papillomatosis?

61 This 3-year-old neutered male Lhasa apso has a 2-week history of a 'disagreeable' odour, which the owners state is coming from the tail area. On physical examination the tail itself is normal, but the perianal area has a swollen, painful area on the right side. A draining tract is located in the centre of the area. The exudate is malodorous, and cytologic examination shows numerous neutrophils, cocci and rods.

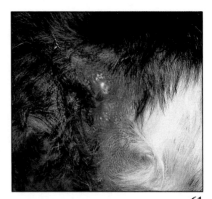

61

(a) What is your most probable diagnosis?
(b) How is this condition best treated?

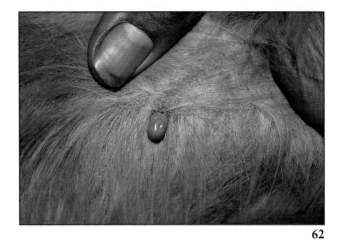

62

62 This canine patient has a tick imbedded in the epidermis of the lateral thoracic area.
(a) What are the cutaneous ramifications of this tick?
(b) What are some common diseases that are tick-transmitted?

63 This 2-year-old spayed female Vizsla has a 2-month history of patchy alopecia which initially involved the head and progressed to involve the trunk. The patient is not pruritic. Skin scrapings and a fungal culture were negative.
(a) What is your tentative diagnosis?
(b) How would you confirm your diagnosis?
(c) Which breeds of dogs have been reported to be predisposed to this dermatologic disease?
(d) What are some of the treatments?

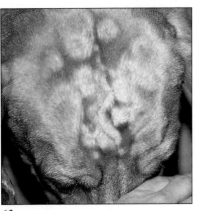
63

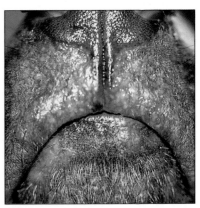
64

64 This 12-year-old mixed-breed dog presented with a several-week history of an ulcerative, painful, non-pruritic skin disease involving mucocutaneous junctions and pressure points. The patient was lethargic and had a decreased appetite. There was no response to a course of broad spectrum antibiotics as well as a course of anti-inflammatory doses of corticosteroids.
(a) What is this uncommon (rare) skin disease of the dog?
(b) How would you make the diagnosis?
(c) What are your differential diagnoses?

65 This elderly female mixed-breed dog was taken to the local humane society because she was found wandering loose in bad weather with numerous open skin 'wounds'. Biopsies were taken for histopathologic examination. Skin scrapings and a fungal culture were negative. A complete blood count and chemistry profile were within normal limits. The patient was bright and alert, eating well and appeared to be in only minor cutaneous discomfort. She was not pruritic, but would occasionally lick her skin lesions.

(a) What is this patient's skin disease?

(b) What is the treatment?

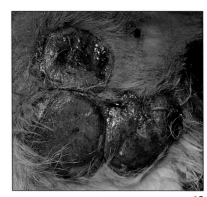

65

66 This 4-year-old male Golden retriever presented with a 3-year history of pruritus involving the feet, face and axillae. The patient also had recurrent otitis externa. The condition was originally seasonal, being most severe at times of high pollen count, but soon became year-round. A diagnosis of allergic inhalant disease (atopy) was made.

(a) List the five most common presenting signs of canine allergic inhalant disease.

(b) What treatment regimes are available?

(c) Are there any specific breed predilections?

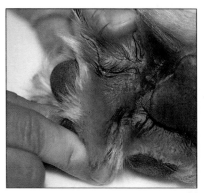

66

67 A middle-aged cat from the state of New Mexico (in the United States) is presented for evaluation with the complaint of fever, depression, lameness and a cough of several months' duration. A solitary ulcerated lesion is present on the trunk, otherwise the skin appears to be normal. Radiographs of the chest show an infiltrative pattern in the lung tissue. Histopathologic examination of the skin lesion shows pyogranulomatous, nodular-to-diffuse inflammation with fungal organisms. The organisms range in size from 10 μ to 80 μ in diameter.
What is the most likely diagnosis?

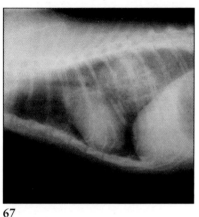 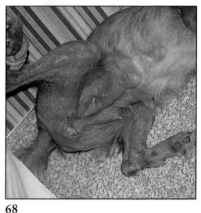

67

68

68 The abdomen of an 8-year-old intact female Golden retriever is pictured. This patient has a history of repeated false pregnancies and irregular oestrous cycles. The skin problem started about 6 months ago with a pruritic erythematous eruption involving the perineal area, perivulvar area and caudal abdomen. The erythema progressed to hyperpigmentation. The owners report that the problem began just after an oestrous cycle and gradually continued to worsen.
(a) What is the most probable diagnosis?
(b) What differential diagnoses would you consider?
(c) How would you make the definitive diagnosis?

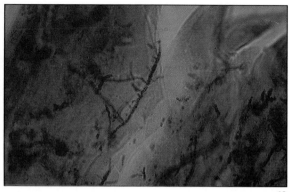

69

69 A 4-year-old female Beagle is presented with a 2-month history of dermatitis characterised by erythematous papules with thick crusts. The lesions are several centimetres in diameter. When the crust of a lesion was removed, a greenish purulent exudate on an oval/round, bleeding, ulcerated surface was found. A direct smear from the surface of this lesion was stained with a Wright-Giemsa stain and revealed the pictured organisms.
(a) What is this organism?
(b) What is the diagnosis and how common is this disease in the dog?
(c) What treatment would you recommend?

70 This rapidly developing, mildly pruritic lesion was found on the foreleg of a 12-year-old American Cocker spaniel. Histopathologic examination revealed a sebaceous adenocarcinoma.
(a) Are these tumours usually solitary or multiple?
(b) Is there a canine breed predilection?
(c) What is the biologic behaviour of these tumours?
(d) What is the most common site of occurrence?

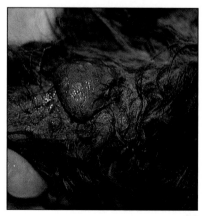

70

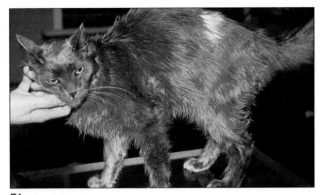

71

71 This 10-year-old neutered male domestic short-haired cat has a 4-month history of a rough, unkempt, greasy-to-the-touch hair coat. The owner reports that the cat's claws are growing at a faster rate than usual. A nodule is palpated on the left side of the ventral neck, in the area of the larynx.
(a) What is the most probable diagnosis?
(b) How would you confirm this?
(c) What is the treatment?

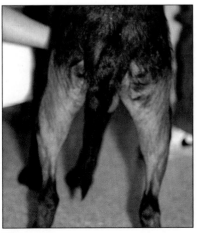

72

72 This 3-year-old male mixed Labrador retriever was neutered several months prior to presentation. The complaint was progressive hair loss, without pruritus, involving the entire trunk and caudal thighs. The hair loss started a few weeks after the neutering. Thyroid tests, as well as a complete blood count and chemistry profile, were within normal limits.
(a) What is the most likely diagnosis?
(b) What is the treatment?

73 This 1-year-old male cat has a 6-month history of follicular plugging, occasional exudation and mild pruritus involving the dorsal, anterior one-third of the tail. Skin scrapings and a fungal culture were negative. There was no evidence of fleas and the cat was strictly an indoor pet.

(a) What is your tentative diagnosis?

(b) What is the treatment?

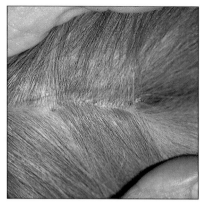

73

74 This middle-aged, black and tan female Dobermann pinscher is presented for evaluation. She was found as a 'stray' in the southeastern portion of the United States. The patient has numerous, exudative lesions and nodules on the head, ears and legs. Skin scrapings were negative for ectoparasites. Cytologic examination of the lesion exudate revealed acute inflammation with neutrophils and eosinophils. Bacterial and fungal cultures were negative. Histopathologic examination of a nodule revealed angiocentric, pyogranulomatous dermatitis with microfilarial segments.

(a) What disease do you suspect?

(b) What additional diagnostic test should be performed to confirm your diagnosis?

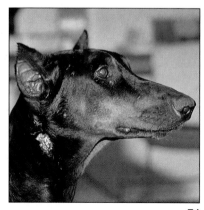

74

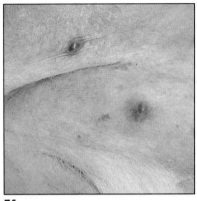

75 Some of the many intradermal nodules found on physical examination of this 9-year-old male Shetland sheepdog are pictured. An anterior abdominal mass was palpated.
(a) What is the diagnosis?
(b) Where is the mass most likely located within the anterior abdomen?
(c) In what other areas are metastatic lesions likely to be found?

75

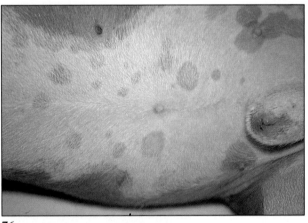

76

76 This young, male intact English bulldog was out in the yard chasing bees. Within 30 minutes, the owners noticed the eruptions seen in this picture.
(a) What is the most probable diagnosis?
(b) What sequela to this event is of grave concern?
(c) Is this skin condition pruritic?

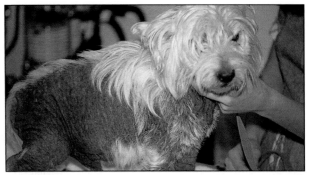

77

77 This 1-year-old West Highland White terrier has an 8-month history of severe pruritus. Physical examination reveals a generalised hyperpigmentation, alopecia, areas of erythema and seborrhoea oleosa (producing a 'greasy feel' to the skin and hair coat). This patient's female litter mate has a similar skin condition.
(a) What is your tentative diagnosis?
(b) What are other differential diagnoses that are important?
(c) How would you confirm the diagnosis?
(d) What is the treatment?

78 This 4-year-old spayed female Golden retriever has a several-month history of a progressively thinning truncal hair coat. The owner reports that she has developed a 'sad' facial expression. A fasting serum chemistry profile is normal except for a high cholesterol value.
(a) What is the most likely diagnosis?
(b) How would you confirm this diagnosis?
(c) What causes the 'sad' expression?

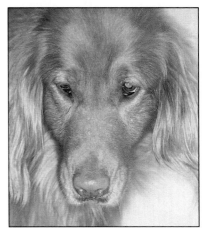

78

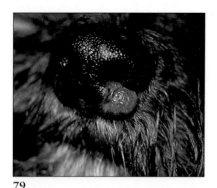

79 An erythematous, ulcerated mass on the ventrolateral aspect of the planum nasale of an 11-year-old, male intact Scottish terrier is pictured. The owners noticed the lesion just a few weeks prior to presentation. -

(a) What is the diagnosis?

(b) What is the biological behaviour of this tumour?

79

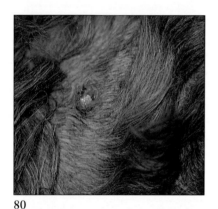

80 This erythematous, ulcerated tumour was found on the left shoulder of a 9-year-old mixed-breed dog. The histopathologic diagnosis is sebaceous adenoma.

(a) Is this a common or rare canine tumour?

(b) What size are these tumours?

(c) Are these tumours solitary or multiple?

80

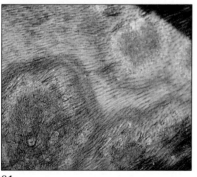

81 This 3-year-old female spayed Labrador retriever had an adverse reaction to an orally administered sulpha-type antibiotic. The histopathologic diagnosis was erythema multiforme.

(a) What other diagnoses would be appropriate based upon the clinical presentation?

(b) How would you treat this patient?

81

82 This 7-year-old Silky terrier presented with an uneven patch of hair loss and hyperpigmentation on the crown of his head. The owner did not know how long the alopecia had been present.
(a) What is the diagnosis?
(b) What is the treatment?

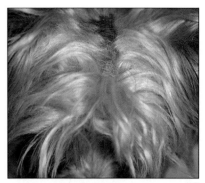

82

83 The face of an 11-month-old female intact Shetland sheepdog with alopecia, erythema, scaling and some hyperpigmentation is pictured. She has atrophy of the temporal muscles. Other clinical signs include similar lesions on her ear pinnae, carpi and tail tip.
(a) What is this disease?
(b) How is the diagnosis made?
(c) What are the two most commonly affected breeds of dog?

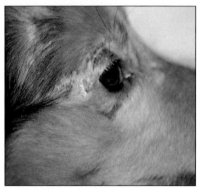

83

84 This 7-year-old, neutered male Pomeranian has a 6-month history of non-pruritic alopecia involving the trunk. The head and legs have a normal hair coat. Thyroid and adrenal function tests were within normal limits. Skin scrapings were negative for demodectic mites.
(a) What are your two main differential diagnoses?
(b) List five breeds of dog that appear to be predisposed to the latter differential diagnosis.

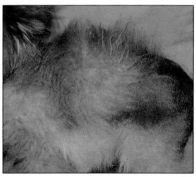

84

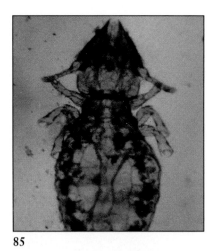

85 A 6-week-old kitten is presented for examination. The owner's major complaint is that the patient is pruritic. Careful examination of the kitten reveals numerous macroscopic parasites (shown).
(a) What is this organism?
(b) What is the best treatment plan?
(c) What important information should be relayed to the owner?

85

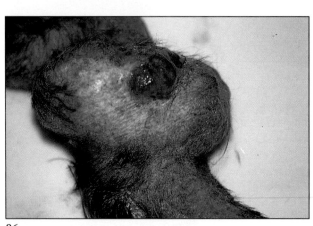

86

86 A mass located on the left forelimb of a 7-year-old mixed-breed dog is pictured. The mass has recurred four times at the same location.
(a) What is your diagnosis?
(b) How is this mass best treated after four unsuccessful attempts at surgical excision?
(c) Are you surprised that the tumour has not metastasized?

87 A cat is presented to you for evaluation of a chronic nasal discharge. Upon physical examination you note a proliferative mass on the nares. Cytologic examination of a smear of the exudate, stained with new methylene blue, reveals active suppurative inflammation and budding yeast.

(a) What is the most likely diagnosis?

(b) What is the treatment?

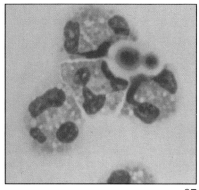

87

88 This 2-year-old American Cocker spaniel presented with a history of numerous cutaneous wounds secondary to normal grooming and combing. Physical examination revealed the skin over the entire trunk to be extremely hyperextensible (**A**). A skin scraping above the left eye resulted in a gaping wound (**B**).

(a) What disease does this patient have?

(b) What is the treatment?

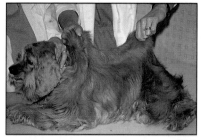

88A

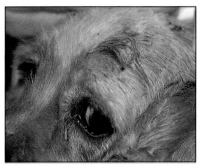

88B

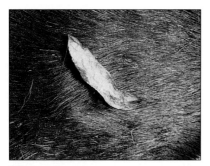

89

89 Shown is an incidental finding on physical examination of a 10-year-old Great Dane. The lesion is firmly attached to the skin and is quite hard.
(a) What is the diagnosis?
(b) How is this lesion best treated?

90 This 6-year-old female white German shepherd dog is presented with a two week history of hypopigmentation of the nose with crusts and erosions extending up the bridge of the nose. Physical examination reveals ulceration of the hard and soft palates, medial aspects of the ear pinnas, vulva and anus. The patient is anorectic, febrile and obviously does not feel well.
(a) What are your three most important differential diagnoses?
(b) What are your three most important diagnostic tests?
(c) What is your diagnosis?
(d) Is the German shepherd dog predisposed?

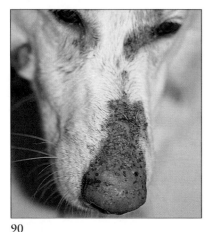

90

91 A recently described heritable neoplastic syndrome in the German shepherd dog (Alsatian) associates the development of multiple dermal fibromas (nodular dermatofibrosis) with the development of two other tumours.
What are these two other tumours?

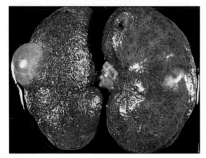

91

92 The skin lesion pictured started as an area of folliculitis. The infection progressed and caused rupture of the hair follicles, producing this larger, raised lesion from which a haemorrhagic-purulent exudate could easily be expressed.
(a) What is this lesion?
(b) What are the three possible aetiologies of this lesion, and which of these is the most common?
(c) Which areas of the body are most likely to be affected with forms of this disease?

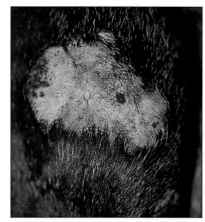

92

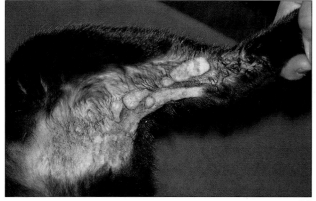

93

93 This cat is presented for intensely pruritic, erythematous, ulcerated lesions on the medial aspect of the left rear leg. The lesions have been recurrent (possibly seasonal) and have been responsive to corticosteroid injections.
(a) What is the most likely diagnosis?
(b) How would you confirm this diagnosis?
(c) What are the underlying etiologies of this condition in the feline?

94 This 9-month-old mixed-breed puppy has a 4-month history of alopecia, erythema and crusts, which have become progressively more severe. The lesions are most severe on the muzzle, periocular areas and pressure points. The patient is non-pruritic. The owners report that he has become less active even though his appetite remains fairly normal. On physical examination (other than the obvious skin disease), a low-grade fever and mild lymphadenopathy are found.

(a) List the six most important differential diagnoses.

(b) What important question about the home care of this patient needs to be asked?

(c) List the three most important diagnostic tests for this patient.

(d) What is the diagnosis?

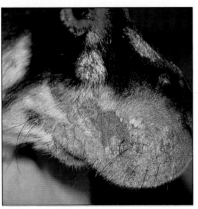
94

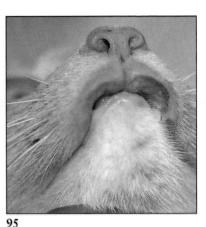
95

95 This 6-year-old domestic short-haired cat is presented for evaluation of the pictured upper lip lesions, which have been recurrent over the past 3 years and have become progressively more severe.

(a) What is the name of this condition?

(b) How would this diagnosis be confirmed?

(c) How would you initially treat this patient?

(d) What are underlying causes in patients with recurrent lesions?

96 This 7-year-old yellow Labrador retriever developed acute erythematous macules and papules which spread peripherally. Some of the lesions had central healing, producing an annular or 'target' pattern. Most of the lesions involved the trunk, but the mucocutaneous junctions were ulcerated. One week before initial development of the skin lesions, the patient received an injection of penicillin for a respiratory infection.

(a) What is the probable diagnosis?

(b) What other differential diagnoses would you consider?

(c) What is the probable cause of the skin disease in this patient?

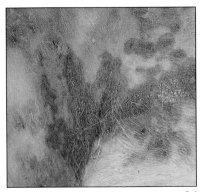
96

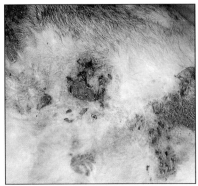
97

97 This middle-aged German shepherd dog presented with a deep pyoderma involving the rump and back. Lesions included a deep folliculitis, furunculosis and a few areas of cellulitis.

(a) What is the most likely diagnosis?

(b) What is (are) the most common bacterial organism(s) associated with this skin disease?

(c) Are these patients usually pruritic?

(d) What is the prognosis for this skin disease?

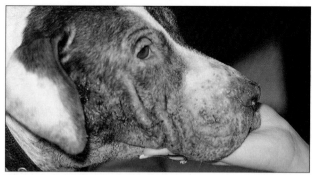

98A

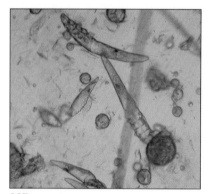

98B

98 This 8-month-old male mixed Pit Bull terrier (**A**) presented with numerous areas of alopecia, erythema, folliculitis and furunculosis. The owners reported that the skin disease was noticed approximately 2 months prior to presentation. The patient is moderately pruritic. Skin scrapings, taken from affected facial skin, feet and trunk, readily reveal this organism (**B**).
(a) What is the diagnosis?
(b) What is your treatment plan?
(c) What important issues must be discussed with the owner?

99 Figures **A** and **B** are the gross- and cross-sections of a solitary mass which was removed from the back of a 3-year-old female spayed miniature Schnauzer.
(a) What is your diagnosis?
(b) What is the biological behaviour of this tumour?

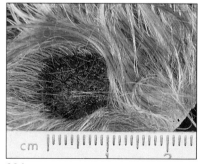

99A

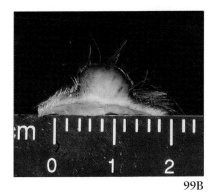
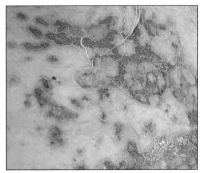

99B

100

100 The abdominal area of a 7-year-old female spayed Shetland sheepdog who was presented with a several-week history of serpiginous ulcerations is pictured. The lesions are mildly pruritic and are apparently painful.
(a) What are your differential diagnoses?
(b) What is the most important diagnostic test?
(c) What is the diagnosis?

101 The feline patient pictured is a breed of cat called the Sphinx. These cats have a very short, downy hair coat that is almost imperceptible to the eye and touch.
(a) How common is this feline breed?
(b) Are there any special maintenance requirements for this breed?

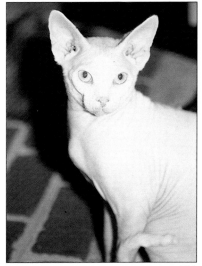

101

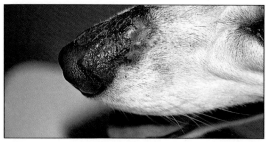

102

102 This 5-year-old German shepherd dog presented with a rapid (few days') onset of folliculitis and furunculosis on the bridge of the nose. The lesion was non-pruritic, but was quite painful. Skin scrapings were negative for demodectic mites. A fungal culture was also negative. The patient had no other cutaneous or systemic abnormalities. This disease is called nasal pyoderma.
(a) Which breeds of dog are most commonly affected with nasal pyoderma?
(b) What other diseases would you consider in your list of differential diagnoses for this patient?
(c) Discuss the important points of the clinical management of this disease.

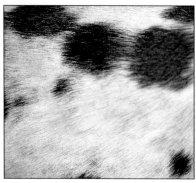

103

103 This Dalmatian presented with patchy alopecia, erythema, coat discolouration and papules involving most of the trunk, but most severely the dorsal trunk. The owners reported mild pruritus, but were most concerned about the cosmetic appearance of their pet. Skin scrapings were negative for demodectic mites.
(a) What are the two most likely diagnoses?
(b) What therapy would you recommend?

104 This 6-month-old domestic short-haired cat is presented for evaluation of non-pruritic, non-painful lesions involving the caudal thighs. (The hair has been clipped to visualise the lesions.) Palpation of the lesions reveals well-circumscribed, raised, firm plaques of a linear configuration. The rest of the physical examination is normal. The owner declines any diagnostic testing.

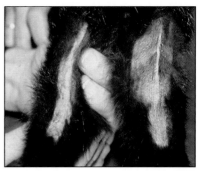

104

(a) What is your clinical diagnosis?
(b) What is the treatment?
(c) If the owner declines treatment, what is the most likely outcome of this condition?

105 A mass on the right rear leg of a 4-year-old dog is pictured. The area has been shaved and prepared for surgical excision. Digital pressure produced a 'dimpling' of the skin, which did not return to normal after 5 minutes. A moderate amount of clear fluid was aspirated. On cytologic evaluation, only a few mature lymphocytes were found.

(a) What is your diagnosis?
(b) How is this tumour best treated?
(c) What is the prognosis for this patient?

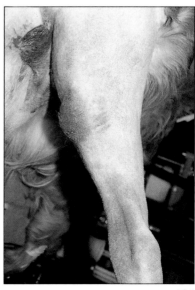

105

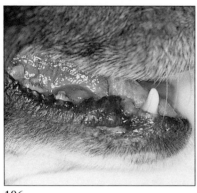

106

106 A mixed Siberian husky developed this erythematous, vegetative mass on the underside of his tongue over the past 6 months. Otherwise, the dog appeared to be quite healthy. The only abnormality in the patient's bloodwork was a mild eosinophilia.
(a) What is the most probable diagnosis?
(b) Is there any canine age, breed and/or sex predilection for the development of this lesion?
(c) What other clinical presentations may be seen with this condition?

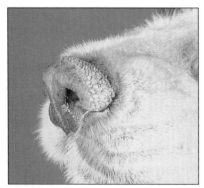

107

107 The nose of a 10-year-old neutered male American Cocker spaniel is shown. The dog is presented for routine examination and vaccinations. The owner states that the dog's nose tissue appears to be excessive and crusty. The duration of the condition is not known. The nose is non-pruritic and non-painful. The rest of the physical examination is normal except for obesity.
(a) What is your diagnosis?
(b) What other areas of the body may be similarly affected?
(c) What is the treatment?
(d) What are the breeds of dogs predisposed to developing this condition?

108 A young, male outdoor cat is presented to you for evaluation of a pruritic skin disease mainly involving the head and feet. A skin scraping taken from the head reveals this mite.
(a) What is this mite?
(b) What is your treatment plan?

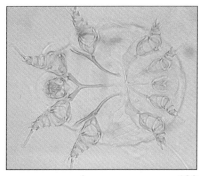

108

109 A mass removed from the external ear canal of a 1-year-old domestic short-haired cat is pictured. The cat was presented to the veterinarian for mild head shaking and pawing at the affected ear.
(a) What is the diagnosis?
(b) What is the site of origin of this mass?
(c) Other than the external ear canal, where else may these lesions be found?

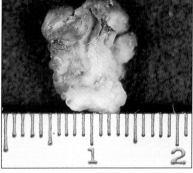

109

110 These intensely pruritic excoriated papules were found on the foot of a young female owner of two dogs. Both dogs had mild rump and tail base pruritus.
(a) What is the most likely diagnosis?
(b) What other differentials should be considered, knowing that the person is exposed to pruritic dogs and no other animals?

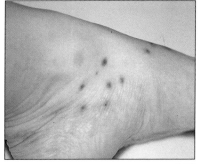

110

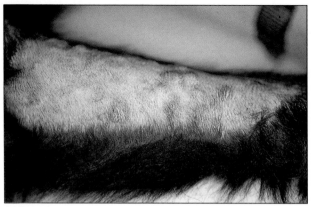

111

111 This 9-year-old male intact black German shepherd dog presented with a several-month history of generalised, pigmented cutaneous nodules which were non-pruritic and not painful. Otherwise, the patient was in very good physical condition, with a normal, complete blood count, chemistry profile and urinalysis.
(a) What is your most important diagnostic test?
(b) What is the diagnosis?
(c) What is the most common internal disease associated with this cutaneous disease?
(d) Is the German shepherd dog predisposed?
(e) What is the treatment?

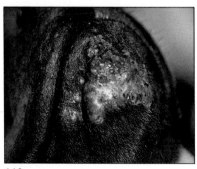

112

112 The chin of a young, mixed Dobermann pinscher with folliculitis, deep folliculitis and furunculosis is shown.
(a) What is the most likely diagnosis?
(b) What are the age, breed, and sex predilections for this cutaneous disease?
(c) What is the recommended therapy for this condition?

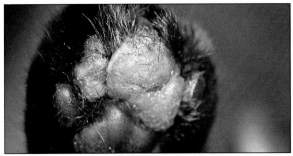

113

113 The forefoot of an 8-year-old indoor cat is shown. Several months ago, the patient developed soft swellings (most non-painful) of multiple footpads involving multiple paws. The surface of some affected pads was cross-hatched with white, scaly stria; others were ulcerated. The patient was lame on the left foreleg. Prescapular lymphadenopathy was evident. Fine needle aspiration cytologic evaluation revealed primarily neutrophils and plasma cells.

(a) What is the probable diagnosis?

(b) How is this diagnosis made?

(c) What is the appropriate therapy?

114 This 8-year-old Pug is presented with numerous flat-topped pustules involving mainly the abdomen and axillary areas. The lesions are non-painful and non-pruritic.

(a) What are your differential diagnoses?

(b) List the most important diagnostic tests.

(c) What is the diagnosis?

(d) How common is this disease in the dog?

(e) Has this disease been reported in the cat?

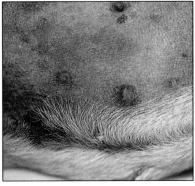

114

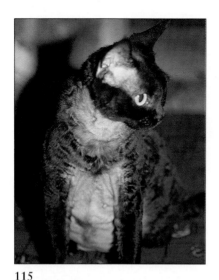

115

115 The feline patient pictured has marked hair loss on the ventral neck, chest, abdomen, caudal thighs and preauricular areas. The patient is non-pruritic.
(a) Which of the following skin problems does this patient have?
1 Self-induced alopecia (i.e. allergic dermatitis). 2 Hormonal hair loss. 3 No skin disease. This is a normal cat.
(b) What breed of cat is this?

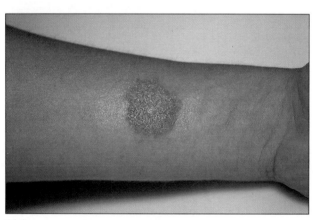

116

116 This slightly raised erythematous lesion was found on the arm of a female veterinary technician. The lesion was solitary and non-pruritic.
(a) What is the most likely diagnosis?
(b) What are likely sources of this infection?

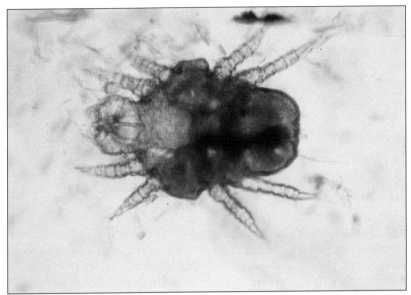

117 You are presented with a very pruritic domestic short-haired indoor cat. The owner reports that her two dogs are also pruritic, but to a lesser degree. Physical examination reveals some areas of self-induced alopecia and a very significant amount of large dandruff flakes. Many skin scrapings are negative for mites. There is no evidence of fleas. A small piece of acetate ('Scotch') tape is used to collect some of the dandruff from the patient's hair coat. This is placed on a slide and examined microscopically. The mite is found. On careful review of the history, the owner reveals that she purchased a rabbit from a local pet shop a few months prior to the onset of the clinical signs in her other pets.

(a) What is the name of the mite pictured?
(b) Is it species specific?
(c) How would you treat this 'case'?
(d) What other information is important for the owner to be aware of?

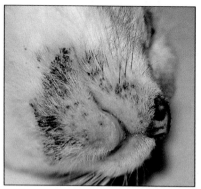

118

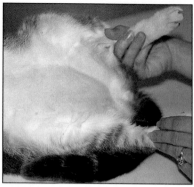

119

118 This 2-year-old female spayed Siamese cat is presented with a 4-month history of partial alopecia, some erythema, crusts and blackheads (comedones) involving the chin and lower lips. The patient is only mildly pruritic. Skin scrapings are negative for demodectic mites, and a fungal culture reveals no growth.
(a) What is your diagnosis?
(b) How would you confirm your diagnosis?

119 This middle-aged female feline is presented for evaluation of hair loss involving the abdominal area. The owner has noticed the progressive hair loss over a 6-month period of time. However, no increased grooming or any form of pruritus has been noticed by the owner. The cat lives indoors and is not exposed to other pets. Microscopic examination of some 'stubbly' hairs plucked from the abdomen reveals normal hair bulbs with frayed ends.
(a) What is your diagnosis?
(b) List four causes of this condition, in order of their prevalence.
(c) What diagnostic tests would you perform on this patient?

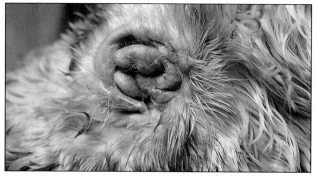

120

120 This blonde American Cocker spaniel is presented for evaluation of a chronic, bilateral otitis. The condition was noticed approximately 4 years ago, and has become progressively more severe. The ears are painful and pruritic, and the owner has noticed a decreased ability of the patient to hear.
(a) What is the clinical diagnosis?
(b) How should this patient be evaluated?
(c) What are the treatment options available?

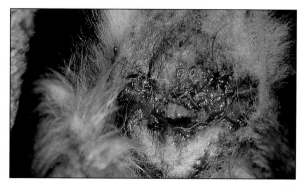

121

121 The perianal area of an older male intact German shepherd dog is shown. List three possible diseases that this clinical slide could represent.

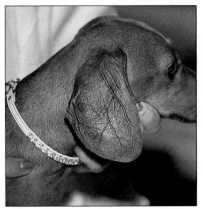

122

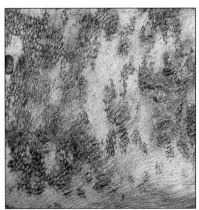

123

122 This 3-year-old female miniature short-hair Dachshund has a 5-month history of bilaterally symmetric alopecia involving the temporal region of the head. Significant alopecia is also noted on the lateral aspects of both ear pinnae. The owners report that the patient is not pruritic. Examination of the external ear canals reveals no abnormalities. Skin scrapings are negative for mites. A fungal culture reveals no significant growth. Bloodwork (a complete blood count and chemistry profile) is within normal limits.
(a) What is your diagnosis?
(b) How would you confirm this diagnosis?
(c) What is the treatment?

123 This 3-year-old female mixed-breed dog developed these hyperpigmented, hyperkeratotic plaques in a symmetrical pattern over the trunk. The lesions were asymptomatic.
(a) What are your differential diagnoses?
(b) How is the diagnosis made?
(c) What is the diagnosis?
(d) What is the treatment?

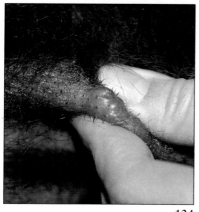

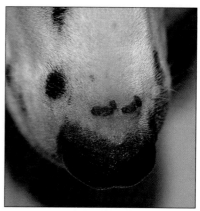

124

125

124 The 10-month-old Chinese Shar pei pictured presented with generalised pitting 'oedema', puffiness and wrinkling of the head and extremities (these characteristics are considered to be normal for this breed). Areas on the ventral neck and in the folds of the forelegs showed small vesicles. When the vesicles were ruptured, a stringy, viscous, clear fluid was evident.
(a) What is this vesicular condition?
(b) What is the clear fluid?
(c) What therapy would you recommend?

125 The owners of this young Dalmatian report that the patient frequently develops sunburn at the junction of the haired and hairless skin of the nose during the warm months of the year. This is the third year the patient has developed this condition. The bridge of the nose is slightly alopecic, erythematous and crusty.
(a) What is the most probable diagnosis?
(b) What is the possible sequela if this condition occurs year after year and the patient's sun exposure is not limited?
(c) If you were unaware of this patient's history, what other skin diseases would you consider?

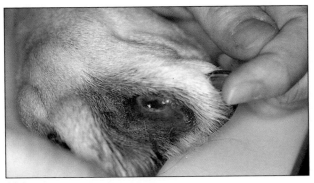

126

126 This 5-year-old Great Dane has a 2-year history of interdigital nodules (cysts). The lesions have progressed to involve all four feet to varying degrees.
(a) What is the diagnosis?
(b) List several underlying conditions that may predispose a canine patient to the development of these lesions.

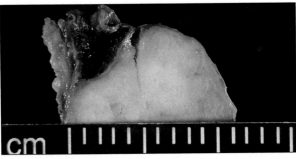

127

127 A 10-year-old female German shepherd dog (Alsatian) presents with a history of polyuria, polydipsia, weakness and difficulty in defecation. Rectal examination reveals a mass, 1.5 cm in diameter, on the ventro-lateral aspect of the anus. A cross-section of the mass is shown.
(a) What is your diagnosis?
(b) How do you account for the clinical signs?

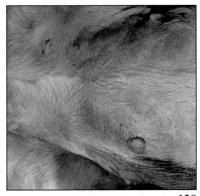

128

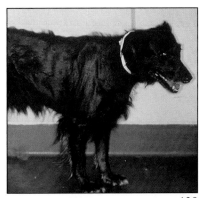

129

128 This 1-year-old Beagle is presented with an 8-month history of non-seasonal skin lesions. The lesions are located primarily on the abdomen, chest and axillae and are quite pruritic. The dog is housed in an outdoor kennel and has a wooden dog house with straw bedding. The patient is not exposed to any other animals. Multiple skin scrapings are negative for mites, but one skin scraping reveals numerous, nematode larvae, 625 – 650 μm in diameter.
(a) What is your diagnosis?
(b) What is your recommended treatment plan?

129 This 8-year-old female spayed mixed-breed dog has a 6-month history of truncal alopecia, generalised seborrhoea sicca, polydipsia, polyuria and pruritus. The patient was diagnosed as having pituitary-dependent hyper-adrenocorticism. What is the cause of the pruritus in this patient, since, in most cases of Cushing's disease, the patient is non-pruritic because of excessive serum cortisol?

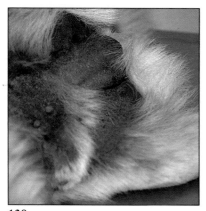

130

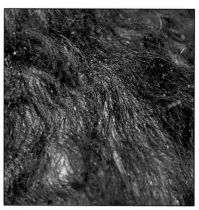

131

130 This 9-year-old male intact mixed Keeshond has a 1-year history of alopecia and hyperpigmentation involving the axillae, abdomen and medial thighs. The owner reports that the patient is not pruritic, and otherwise appears to be in very good health. However, the owner did (embarrassingly) mention that her neighbour's intact male dog has recently been sexually attracted to her dog. Other than the obvious skin changes, the only other abnormality noted on physical examination was that the left testicle was markedly larger and firmer than the right testicle.
(a) What is your diagnosis?
(b) What is the appropriate therapy?
(c) What precautions should be taken prior to therapy?

131 This 5-year-old female Standard Poodle has a long history of excessive scaling which progressed to a noticeably abnormal hair coat. Physical examination reveals that the scales are tightly adhered to the skin and hairs, and appear as thick crusts. The owner reports that the patient is mildly–to–non-pruritic. Routine, diagnostic, dermatologic tests are negative or within normal limits.
(a) What is your most likely diagnosis?
(b) How would you confirm this diagnosis?
(c) What is the treatment?

132 A young male intact Akita is presented with a several-month history of skin disease which was first noticed on the face and progressed to the legs and scrotum.
(a) What is your most likely diagnosis?
(b) How would you confirm this diagnosis?

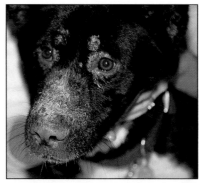

132

133 This young male neutered miniature Schnauzer presented with a several-month history of non-pruritic hair loss in a bilaterally symmetric pattern over the lateral thoraco-lumbar areas.
(a) What are your differential diagnoses?
(b) What is the diagnosis?
(c) What other breeds have a similar (hereditary?) cutaneous disease?

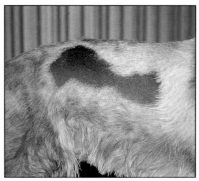

133

134 The standard short-haired Dachshund pictured has primary acanthosis nigricans.
(a) How common is this disease?
(b) What is the age of onset?
(c) Which breed(s) is/are involved?

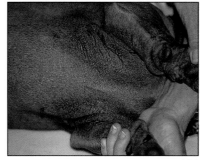

134

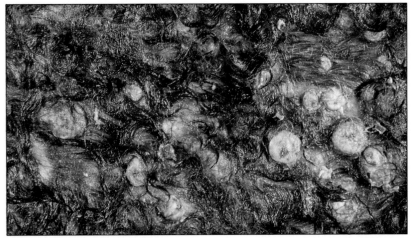

135

135 A few of the many masses found on physical examination of this 5-year-old female spayed Scottish terrier are pictured. Several of the masses were removed and submitted for histopathologic examination. A portion of the histopathology report stated that 'there are numerous intra-epidermal Pautrier microabscesses'.
(a) What is the diagnosis?
(b) What is a 'Pautrier microabscess'?

136 You are requested to make a 'house call' to a kennel in midsummer because the owner is concerned that many of his hunting dogs are chewing their feet. When you examine the premises, you observe that the dogs are housed in individual runs and houses, but share a common exercise pen. The floors of the runs are gravel, and are rinsed daily with water. No chemicals are used. The exercise pen is grass-covered and the faeces are removed weekly. The dogs all have similar lesions, to varying degrees, on their footpads and interdigital areas (**A**). Otherwise, the dogs all appear to be healthy except for the observation of an occasional, loose, bloody stool. In addition to the above, one of the kennel helpers has complained of intensely itchy feet (**B**).
(a) What is the most likely diagnosis?
(b) What are your treatment recommendations?

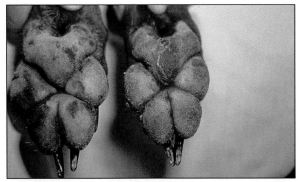

136A

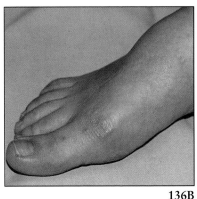

136B

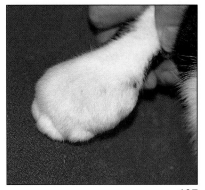

137

137 The swollen forefoot of a 13-year-old domestic short-haired cat is pictured (**137**). The owner has noticed the foot gradually enlarging over the past 3 weeks. On examination the foot is not painful, and there are no clinical signs associated with inflammation, such as erythema and increased warmth. On palpation the foot is soft, but not oedematous. The regional lymph nodes are normal.

(a) What is this tumour?

(b) List two other differential diagnoses.

(c) If you aspirate the mass, what would you find on cytologic examination of the stained aspirate?

(d) Why is the mass so soft?

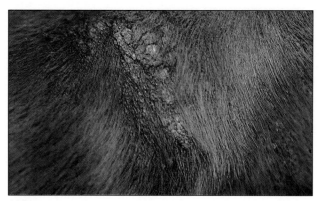

138

138 This 6-year-old blonde male intact American Cocker spaniel has a several-year history of a progressive skin disease. Physical examination reveals diffuse follicular plugging with hyperkeratotic fronds, seen associated with the affected hair follicles. Skin scrapings and a fungal culture are negative. Thyroid function tests are within normal limits. Skin biopsies submitted for histopathologic examination in 10% buffered formalin show disproportionately marked (in comparison to the surface of the epidermis) hair follicular orthokeratotic hyperkeratosis.
(a) What is your diagnosis?
(b) What is the treatment?

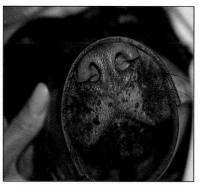

139

139 This 2-year-old Rottweiler presented with a several-month history of a progressive loss of pigment of the nose and periocular areas. The owners also noticed a few white patches where black hair used to be.
(a) What is the clinical diagnosis for the condition described?
(b) Which breeds of dogs appear to be predisposed?

140 A culture taken from this English bulldog's interdigital lesion failed to grow any bacteria. Skin scrapings for demodectic mites were negative. A diagnosis of sterile pyogranulomas or interdigital cysts was made.
(a) Which breeds of dog are most likely to develop this disease?
(b) What is the treatment of choice?

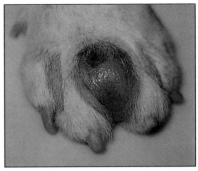

140

141 Pictured is an ulcerated lesion on the nose of an elderly white domestic short-haired cat. This cat has spent most of his life outdoors. Other than the nose lesion, he is quite healthy.
(a) What is your diagnosis?
(b) What factor probably contributed to the development of this lesion in this patient?

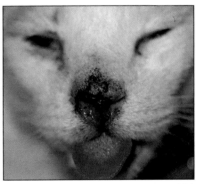

141

142 This young male cat is presented for evaluation. The owner reported that approximately 1 week ago the cat had been accidentally left outside all night in sub-freezing temperatures. Physical examination finds the ear pinnae to be sensitive to the touch. The tips of the pinnae are erythematous with areas of necrosis.
(a) What is the diagnosis?
(b) What is the treatment?

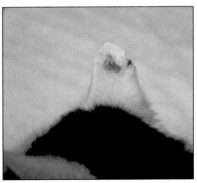

142

143 This 9-year-old neutered male cat has a 2-year history of erythema, seborrhoea oleosa, crusting, partial alopecia and occasional exudation over the anterior, cranial one-third of the tail. The owner reports mild pruritus. Skin scrapings and a fungal culture were negative, and no evidence of fleas was found after very careful examination.
(a) What is your most likely diagnosis?
(b) How would you confirm this diagnosis?
(c) What is the treatment?

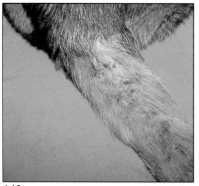

143

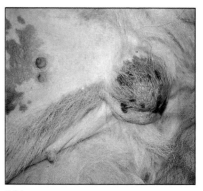

144

144 The abdomen, prepuce and scrotum of an 11-year-old intact male mixed-breed dog is pictured. The patient was presented for routine examination and vaccination; however, the veterinarian noticed a line of erythema extending from the scrotum up the middle of the prepuce. Testicular palpation revealed that the left testicle was significantly larger than the right testicle.
(a) What is the name given to the skin change noted on this patient's abdomen?
(b) Which disease is it associated with?

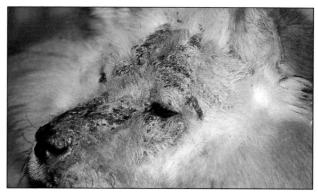

145

145 This 3-year-old female spayed Chow Chow is presented with a 7-week history of alopecia, crusts, erosions and ulcerations involving the face and legs. Owners report that she is mildly pruritic and somewhat painful. A 4-week course of an 'appropriate' antibiotic was not helpful, and the lesions continued to progress.
(a) What is your list of differential diagnoses?
(b) Which diagnostic tests are most important?
(c) What is the diagnosis?
(d) Is this disease curable?
(e) Is this disease treatable?
(f) List drugs commonly used for treatment.

146 This 5-year-old female spayed Golden retriever created these ulcerated, indurated lesions over her carpal areas every year when the pollen count was very high. She also had seasonal otitis externa and interdigital erythema.
(a) What is the common name of this self-induced cutaneous disease?
(b) What is the underlying etiology in this particular patient?

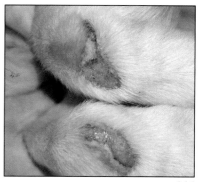

146

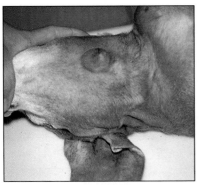

147

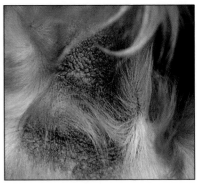

148

147 A 'pigmented' tumour on the ventral neck of an elderly female short-haired Dachshund is pictured. The owner had noticed the lesion 6 months prior to presentation, and stated that it was slowly increasing in size. The tumour was non-pruritic and not painful.
(a) What are your differential diagnoses?
(b) How would you confirm your diagnosis?
(c) How would you treat this tumour?
(d) What is the prognosis for this type of tumour in the dog?

148 The hyperpigmented, lichenified, seborrhoeic axillary area of a 6-year-old Golden retriever with allergic inhalant disease (atopy) is pictured.
(a) What is the term used to describe these cutaneous axillary changes?
(b) Other than allergic inhalant disease, what primary skin diseases can lead to these changes?

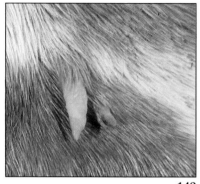

149

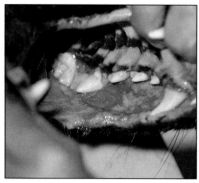

150

149 This 9-year-old Basset hound was presented for examination of a lesion that was noticed on the hindlimb several months previously and appeared to be increasing in size. The lesion did not bother the patient but was of concern to the patient's owners.

(a) What is the diagnosis?

(b) What are other terms used to describe this lesion?

(c) What is the biologic behaviour of this lesion?

150 This 8-year-old male German shepherd dog presented with a several-week history of ulcerations of the lips, nose and oral mucosa, as well on the scrotum and anus. The footpads were sloughing, and the patient was quite painful, anorectic and febrile.

(a) List possible differential diagnoses.

(b) What laboratory testing is indicated?

(c) What is the diagnosis?

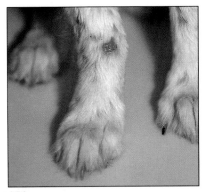

151

151 The right foreleg of a 9-month-old Shetland sheepdog with canine familial dermatomyositis is pictured. The patient has similar lesions on the face, ear pinnae, tail tip and numerous pressure points.
(a) Are the Shetland sheepdog and collie the only breeds of dog reported to have this disease?
(b) What is the aetiopathogenesis of this disease?
(c) What is the treatment?

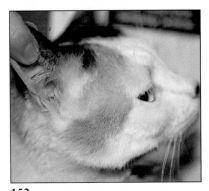

152

152 This 7-year-old female spayed domestic short-haired cat was presented with a complaint of thinning of the hair in the area just anterior to the ear base. The owner did not know how long this condition had existed. There was no evidence or history of pruritus.
(a) Does this cat have a 'skin disease'?
(b) What is this condition called?

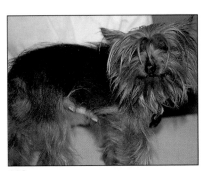

153

153 This 18-month-old Yorkshire terrier presented with a history of thin, stubbly hairs involving the black coat only. The tan-coloured hairs were normal. There was no pruritus and no other evidence of skin disease.
(a) What is the diagnosis?
(b) How is the diagnosis made?
(c) What is the treatment?

154 This 7-year-old neutered male Labrador retriever cross was presented for evaluation of recent skin lesions over the entire dorsal trunk. The patient had a long history of 'allergies', and had been receiving 0.5 – 1.0 mg/kg of prednisone every 48 hours for the past few years. Physical examination reveals large 'encrusted' plaques along the entire dorsum. On palpation, the plaques are very hard and stone-like.

(a) What is your most likely diagnosis?

(b) How would you confirm this diagnosis?

(c) How would you treat this patient?

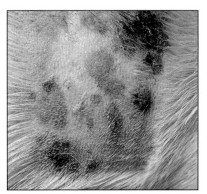

154

155 This young male neutered domestic short-haired cat developed facial excoriations each summer and autumn when he was infested with fleas.

(a) What are other presenting clinical signs of feline flea bite hypersensitivity?

(b) What is the treatment?

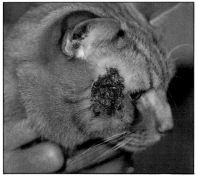

155

156 This 6-year-old female spayed mixed collie presented with nasal depigmentation of 2 months' duration. No other cutaneous or systemic abnormalities were observed.

(a) What are your differential diagnoses?

(b) What is the most important diagnostic test?

(c) What is the diagnosis?

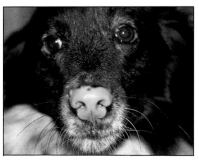

156

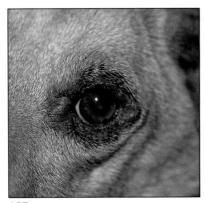

157

157 This 5-year-old mixed-breed dog was being intradermally allergy tested for allergic inhalant disease (atopy), without sedation, when the technician noticed swelling of the periocular areas followed by difficult respiration.
(a) What is the clinical cutaneous diagnosis?
(b) What is the 'systemic' diagnosis?
(c) How common is this response to intradermally injected skin test antigens?
(d) What would be a future concern in this particular patient?

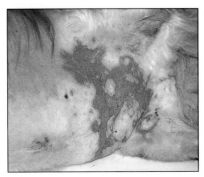

158

158 This middle-aged male neutered Shetland sheepdog is presented with a several-month history of ulcerative lesions involving the axillary areas, abdomen and inguinal area. Antibiotics and low-dose cortico-steroids have been of minimal benefit.
(a) What are your differential diagnoses?
(b) What is the diagnosis?

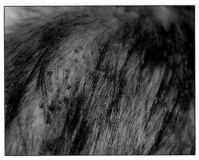

159

159 The rump of a young male neutered cat is pictured. The major complaint mentioned by the owner is intense itching with thinning of the hair coat. Close examination reveals excoriated papules. This condition in the feline patient is termed 'milliary dermatitis'. List the numerous causes of feline milliary dermatitis in order of their 'importance'.

160 The abdomen of a 22-year-old female who recently purchased a cat from a local pet shop is pictured. The cat appeared to be normal except for an excessive, fine white scale over his entire body. The owner reported that the cat was not pruritic. The owner's intensely pruritic papules were present on her abdomen and along her 'bra' line. What is most likely causing this owner's intense discomfort?

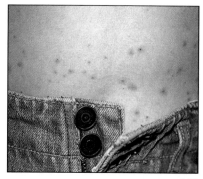

160

161 The forefoot of a 5-year-old female spayed Shetland sheepdog mix is pictured. This patient has had allergic inhalant disease (atopy) since 9 months of age. Hyposensitization injections (immunotherapy) were of little benefit, and antihistamines were not helpful. Her discomfort was controlled on relatively high doses of oral corticosteroids. She was presented with a 'flare-up' of her skin disease, which mainly involved her face and feet; however, numerous erythematous patches were found on her trunk.

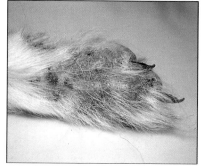

161

(a) What are your major differential diagnoses?
(b) Why is treatment of this patient so difficult?

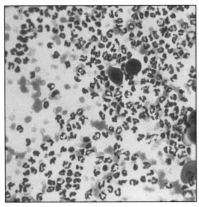

162

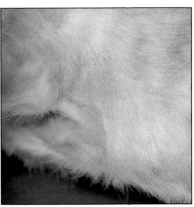

163

162 A 10-year-old mixed-breed cat is presented to you for evaluation of paronychia (nail bed inflammation). All of the digits are affected. Physical examination reveals a thick, greenish discharge from the nail bed. The toes are quite painful. General skin evaluation reveals diffuse scaling and crusting, as well as thinning of the hair coat. The medial aspects of the ear pinnae are erythematous, and small, intact pustules, as well as crusts, are observed. Material collected from the nail bed exudate, stained and microscopically examined, reveals the cells pictured.
(a) What is the most likely diagnosis?
(b) What are the cells seen?
(c) How is this diagnosis confirmed?

163 This 9-year-old female spayed female domestic short-haired cat presented with a several-month history of cutaneous erythema and mild hair loss. Physical examination revealed a thin cat with marked, generalised erythroderma and several palpable cutaneous (epidermal) nodules.
(a) What is the most likely diagnosis?
(b) How would you confirm this diagnosis?
(c) Where may you expect to find metastatic disease?

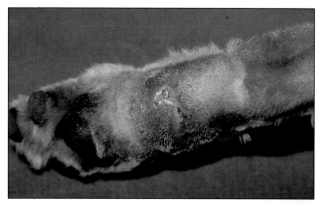

164A

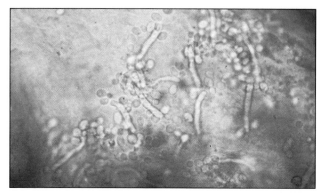

164B

164 This middle-aged male mixed-breed dog is presented for evaluation of a painful, swollen, non-healing wound on the right foreleg (**A**). A skin biopsy was taken and submitted for histopathologic examination. Samples for bacterial and fungal cultures were also obtained. The skin biopsy revealed a diffuse pyogranulomatous infiltrate with fungal organisms. The fungal culture grew *Prototheca wickerhammi* (**B**). The bacterial culture was negative.

(a) What is the source of this infection?

(b) What other organs may be involved?

(c) Is this disease considered to be of zoonotic importance?

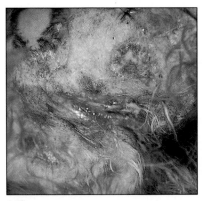

165

165 This 5-year-old Yorkshire terrier is presented with a 2-month history of painful ulcerations of the abdomen and inguinal areas. She is febrile and anorectic. An appropriate course of antibiotics has not been helpful.
(a) What are your differential diagnoses?
(b) What is the diagnosis?
(c) Is this a common disease?
(d) Is the Yorkshire terrier predisposed?

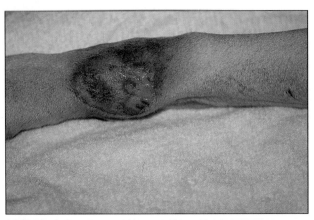

166

166 The foreleg of a 9-year-old female Great Dane is pictured. The owners report that she has been constantly chewing the right carpal area for the past 2 months. She has developed a mild but apparent lameness in this leg. There are no other skin lesions. Radiographs show lytic and proliferative changes in the metaphyseal region of the radius.
(a) What is this skin disease called?
(b) What is the underlying cause in this patient?
(c) List other possible causes of this self-induced leg trauma.

167 The preauricular area of an 11-year-old domestic short-haired cat is pictured. The owner noticed that the area was becoming alopecic, and also noticed the development of raised, hyper-pigmented plaques. List four possible differential diagnoses.

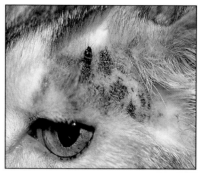

167

168 This 6-year-old male Golden retriever has a several-year history of allergic inhalant disease (atopy) which had been well controlled by hyposensitization injections (immunotherapy) and the occasional use of oral corticosteroids for flare-ups. Several weeks after the patient had been boarded at a local, reputable kennel, he became intensely pruritic, with no response to increasing levels of cortico-steroids. On presentation, the patient had crusting of the ear pinnal margins, elbows and hocks. He also had an intensely pruritic papular dermatitis involving the abdomen and chest (**A, B**).

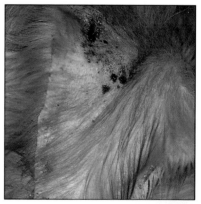

168A

(a) What is the diagnosis?
(b) How is the diagnosis made?
(c) What is the treatment?
(d) How can this disease be contracted?
(e) Is this a zoonotic disease?

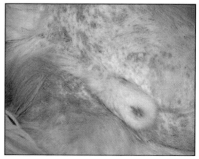

168B

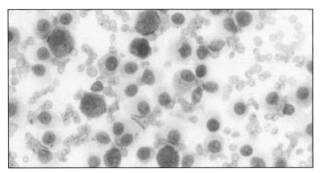

169

169 An 11-year-old cat is presented with a 1.7 cm-wide, slightly raised, moderately pruritic, firm, indurated mass on the neck. The owner noticed the mass approximately 1 year prior to presentation. The mass was non-painful and non-pruritic. A fine needle aspirate of the mass, stained and microscopically examined, revealed the cells pictured.
(a) What is your diagnosis?
(b) How would you treat this patient?

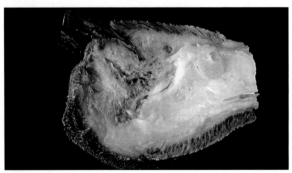

170

170 The cross-section of a tumour surgically removed from the digit of a 9-year-old Standard Poodle is pictured.
(a) What is the diagnosis?
(b) What is the primary differential diagnosis?
(c) What is the prognosis?

171 This 9-year-old domestic short-haired cat developed these asymmetric plaque-like lesions on the face and head 2 months prior to presentation. The lesions are non-pruritic. A repositol corticosteroid injection caused transient worsening of the lesions. Biopsy and histopathologic examination of the lesion revealed a neutrophilic peri-folliculitis and epidermitis.

(a) What is the most likely diagnosis?

(b) What is the usual aetiologic agent?

(c) What is the appropriate therapy?

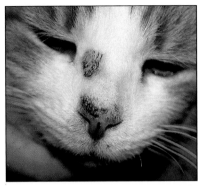

171

172 The cat pictured has a 3-year history of an intense, non-seasonal pruritic dermatitis involving the head and neck. The pruritus was partially responsive to glucocorti-coids. Skin scrapings, dermatophyte culture and intradermal skin testing for allergic inhalant disease were all negative.

(a) What is the most probable diagnosis?

(b) How is this diagnosis made?

(c) What are other possible clinical presentations of this disease in the cat?

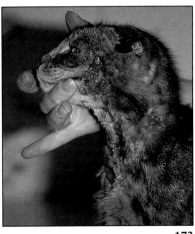

172

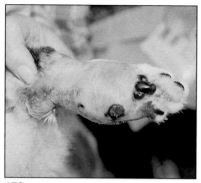

173

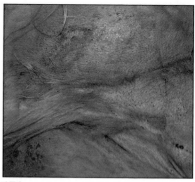

174

173 This cat is presented to you for evaluation of severe swelling of the foot. The lesion has been present for greater than 1 month. Examination reveals a painful, swollen foot that is cold to the touch. There are multiple draining fistulas and hard, yellow, 2 – 5 mm granules are visible in the debris.
(a) What is the most likely diagnosis?
(b) Which diagnostic tests would you perform to confirm the diagnosis?
(c) What are the treatment options?

174 A 1-year-old mixed Golden retriever had relatively normal skin until she was professionally clipped, bathed, dipped and given a 'hot oil' treatment at the groomers. About 24 – 48 hours after the 'grooming', the owners noticed considerable pruritus and the development of this erythematous rash. Upon questioning the groomers, it was learned that other dogs treated in this fashion had not developed skin lesions.
(a) What is the most likely diagnosis?
(b) What type of immunologic response is responsible for this form of cutaneous reaction?
(c) What therapy would you recommend?

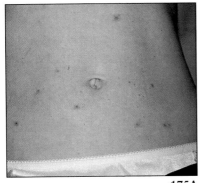

175A

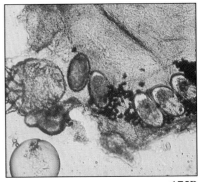

175B

175 A mixed-breed 4-month-old puppy was adopted from a local animal shelter. The pup was presented to his veterinarian for physical examination and vaccination. No abnormalities were found, except for a positive faecal flotation for roundworm ova, for which treatment was dispensed. Several weeks later, the pup started to scratch and the pruritus accellerated over the next few weeks to the point where the pup was up all night scratching. The patient was re-presented to the local veterinarian for evaluation of the pruritus. In reviewing the history (extremely important!), it was learned that the owner had intensely pruritic papules on her abdomen (**A**) and along her 'bra' line. Many skin scrapings were performed on the canine patient and, after exhaustive scrapings, a *Sarcoptes scabiei* mite was found. (**B**) shows the burrow (with eggs and faeces) of a canine scabies mite in human skin.

(a) Is this disease contagious to humans?
(b) Do the mites live in the environment?
(c) What is the appropriate treatment for the canine patient?
(d) What is the treatment for the human owner?

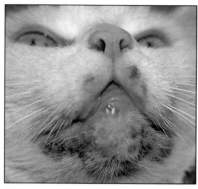

176

176 This 5-year-old domestic short-haired cat has a 2-year history of erythema, comedones, and mild pruritus associated with the chin area. Skin scrapings are negative for demodectic mites, and a fungal culture reveals no significant growth. The rest of the physical examination is within normal limits.
(a) What is your most likely diagnosis?
(b) What are the possible underlying causes (in order of importance) of this feline disease?
(c) How is this disease diagnosed?
(d) What is the therapy?

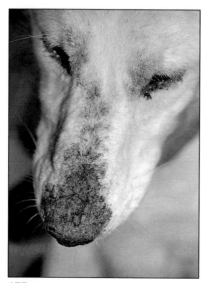

177

177 This 2-year-old female intact German shepherd dog has a several-month history of muzzle and periocular dermatitis. The lesions are encrusted, erythematous, non-pruritic and mildly painful. Similar lesions are noted on the hocks, elbows and other pressure points. The patient is fed a well-balanced commercial dog food. Skin scrapings were negative, and a fungal culture showed no significant growth.
(a) What are your major differential diagnoses?
(b) What is the diagnosis?
(c) How would you confirm this?
(d) What is the treatment?

178 Pictured here are the gross-(**A**) and cross-sections (**B**) of a mass removed from the perianal area of an 8-year-old male intact black Labrador retriever.
(a) What is your diagnosis?
(b) How is this tumour best treated?
(c) What other recommendations would you give to the owner to prevent other similar tumours from arising in this area?

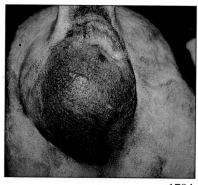

178A

179 This 12-year-old domestic short-haired cat presented with alopecia, erythema, crusts and erosions involving mainly the muzzle and feet. A purulent exudate was present around the nail beds. Several erythematous plaques were noted on the abdomen.
(a) List four possible differential diagnoses.
(b) List three of the most important diagnostic tests.

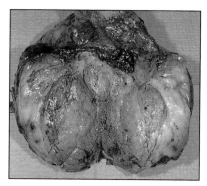

178B

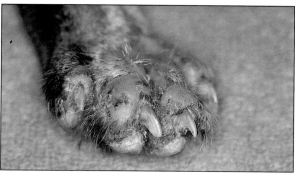

179

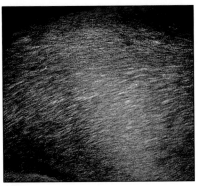

180

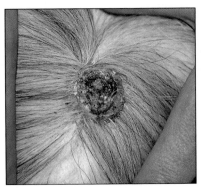

181

180 The lateral thoracic area of a 2-year-old female intact blue and rust Dobermann pinscher is pictured. The owner reports that the patient had a normal coat until approximately 1 year of age. At that time the truncal coat started to become sparse, and the owner noted 'dandruff' (seborrhoea sicca). The patient was non-pruritic. Skin scrapings were negative for demodectic mites, and thyroid function tests were normal.

(a) What skin disease does this patient have?

(b) What are the typical clinical signs and/or secondary skin problems associated with this disease?

(c) What is the treatment?

181 This 7-year-old Norwegian elkhound presented with numerous ulcerated lesions on the trunk. The histopathologic diagnosis is keratoacanthoma (intracutaneous cornifying epithelioma).

(a) What is the biologic behaviour of these lesions?

(b) Which two canine breeds are definitely predisposed to the development of multiple keratoacanthomas?

182 The bruise on the chest of this 4-year-old miniature Schnauzer was noticed by the owner after the patient was professionally groomed. After questioning the groomer, it was learned that the dog jumped off the grooming table and fell.
(a) If this patient were presented to you, what would your major concern be?
(b) What underlying systemic diseases would you consider?

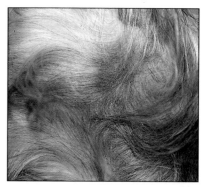

182

183 Full thickness epidermal sloughing involving a large area of the trunk of a 4-year-old Rottweiler is shown. The patient's oral mucosa was also involved. The diagnosis is toxic epidermal necrolysis.
(a) List other possible differential diagnoses for this clinical presentation.
(b) What are the major possible causes?

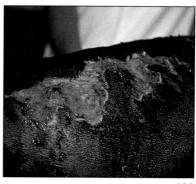

183

184 This eroded, crusted lesion on a pressure point on the rear leg of an 11-year-old spayed female mixed-breed dog is due to superficial necrolytic dermatitis.
(a) What are some possible underlying causes of this disease?
(b) What is the treatment?

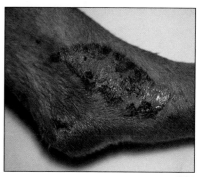

184

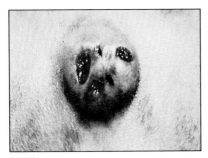

185A

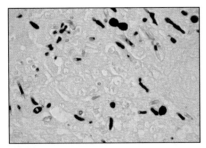

185B

185 A middle-aged male neutered outdoor cat is presented for evaluation of a slowly developing subcutaneous nodule on his thorax. Examination of the lesion reveals an ulcerated, non-painful, cool mass (**A**). The lesion was excised and portions submitted for histopathology, bacterial culture and fungal culture. The bacterial culture was negative. The fungal culture revealed a significant growth of *Drechslera* spp. A section of the histopathologic specimen is shown (**B**).
(a) What is your diagnosis?
(b) What are available treatment options?
(c) What is the prognosis for this patient?

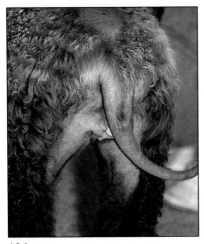

186

186 This 3-year-old female intact Irish water spaniel presented with a several-month history of progressive, non-pruritic, hair loss involving the caudal thighs, perineum, tail, rump, lateral thoracic areas and neck. A complete blood count, chemistry profile and thyroid tests were within normal limits. Her oestrous cycles had been normal, with no history of false pregnancies.
(a) What is the most probable diagnosis?
(b) How is this diagnosis confirmed?
(c) What is the treatment?

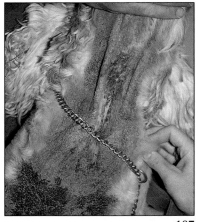

187

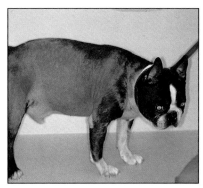

188

187 This 6-year-old male neutered American Cocker spaniel has a 3-year history of a generalised greasy seborrhoea. The most severely involved areas are the ears, ventral neck, axillae and abdomen. There is marked alopecia, hyperpigmentation with lichenification and an adherent, greasy, sebaceous deposit on the affected skin. The owner reports moderate pruritus. Skin scrapings are negative for mites. A fungal culture reveals no significant growth. Skin cytology shows numerous cocci and yeast (*Malassezia*). A complete blood count and chemistry profile are normal.
(a) What is your tentative diagnosis?
(b) How would you confirm this?
(c) What is the treatment?

188 This 6-year-old male neutered Boston terrier is presented for evaluation. The patient has significant truncal hair loss which the owner reports has been present for several months. The owner also reports that the dog's water consumption has tripled and that he is urinating in the house. Physical examination reveals a very thin truncal hair coat. The skin itself is quite thin, which is best seen on the abdomen. In this area the skin thinness allows for visualisation of the cutaneous abdominal vasculature.
(a) What is the most likely diagnosis?
(b) How would you confirm your diagnosis?
(c) What is the treatment?
(d) Are there any known breed pre-dispositions?

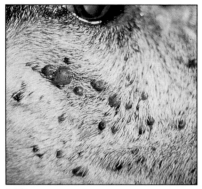

189 Some of the many lesions on the face of a 13-year-old mixed-breed dog are pictured. The owner reports that they have been developing over the last 2 years. They are non-pruritic and do not bother the dog in any way. The owner was a bit concerned about the cosmetic appearance of these multiple lesions.

(a) What are these lesions?
(b) What is the possible aetiology?

189

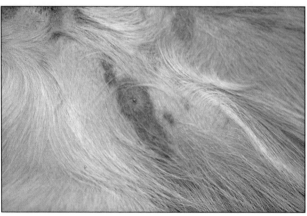

190

190 This middle-aged dog presented with lesions on the chest, abdomen, medial thighs and hindlimbs. The owners reported that the lesions were intensely pruritic. Upon close physical examination, the lesions were found to be primarily erythematous pustules and haemorrhagic bullae. Cytology of the lesions revealed neutrophils, occasional eosinophils and coccoid, paired bacteria.

(a) What is the most likely diagnosis?
(b) What is/are the probable causative organism(s)?
(c) List several differential diagnoses.

191 The dorsal neck of a 2-year-old Airedale terrier is shown. These intensely pruritic, erythematous lesions developed around the neck 2 weeks after the owner placed a new flea collar on the pet.
(a) What is the diagnosis?
(b) How is this condition best treated?
(c) How can this condition be prevented?

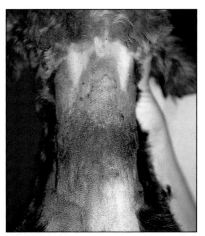

191

192 This pigmented, nodular tumour was found on the forefoot of a 10-year-old Yorkshire terrier. The histopathologic diagnosis is neuroendocrine tumour (Merkel cell tumour).
(a) Is this tumour benign or malignant?
(b) What are the most common sites of occurrence?

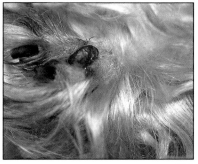

192

193 A young male outdoor cat is presented for evaluation of a non-healing facial wound of several months' duration. A stained impression smear of the exudate reveals these intracellular organisms.
(a) What is the diagnosis?
(b) What are the treatment options?
(c) What education would you provide the owner?

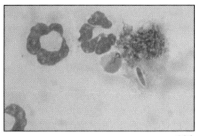

193

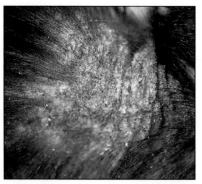

194 A 9-year-old domestic short-haired cat presenting with 'seborrhoea' of unknown aetiology is shown. Physical examination reveals a thin patient with extensive epidermal scale and exfoliation, erythema and hair loss. Skin biopsies for histopathologic examination and an antinuclear antibody (ANA) test are consistent with systemic lupus erythematous. List some other causes for this feline cutaneous presentation.

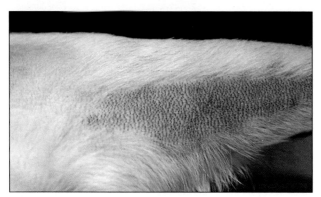

195

195 This 14-month-old female intact Pug was presented because the owner noticed some black spots and darkening of the skin on the medial aspect of the left rear leg. The rest of the patient's skin appeared to be normal. The owner reported that the dog did not bother the lesion in any way and otherwise was quite healthy.
(a) What is the most important diagnostic test to perform, given the age of the dog and appearance of the lesion?
(b) What would you find?
(c) How is this disease treated?
(d) Is this a hereditary disease?

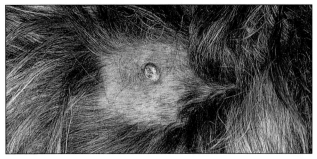

196

196 One of several masses arising on the back of an 8-year-old Yorkshire terrier is pictured. On careful clinical examination, a small pore was found in the centre of the mass. On applying gentle, digital pressure, a small amount of grey/tan, slightly oily material was expressed from the mass onto the skin surface.
(a) List the two major differential diagnoses.
(b) What is the material that has been extruded through the pore?
(c) How are these lesions best treated?
(d) What could be the consequence if the mass were squeezed very firmly?
(e) Which breed of dog is predisposed to developing this condition?

197 This feline patient developed papulo-pustular, coalescing lesions involving the entire trunk, 9 months after initiation of injectable gold salt therapy for pemphigus foliaceous. (The patient's pemphigus foliaceous had been well controlled on the gold salt therapy.)
(a) What are your two major differential diagnoses?
(b) What is the most important diagnostic test?
(c) How would you now treat this patient's pemphigus foliaceous?

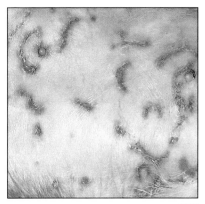

197

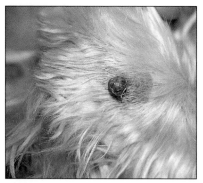

198

198 This 14-year-old West Highland White terrier presented for evaluation of numerous 'growths'. The lesion pictured is on the lateral aspect of the left ear pinna. Histopathologic examination reveals a cutaneous papilloma.
(a) Are these lesions benign or malignant?
(b) Are they usually solitary or multiple?
(c) What is their clinical significance?

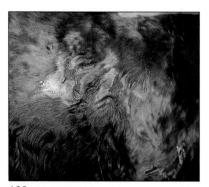

199

199 This American Cocker spaniel was presented to his veterinarian 1 week after being professionally groomed and bathed. The owners noticed pain, then swelling, over the right shoulder area. Apparently, a scab formed, which fell off, leaving the lesion shown.
(a) What is the diagnosis?
(b) What is the most significant sequela to this type of skin trauma?

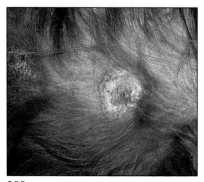

200

200 The 'end-stage' lesion seen on a dog with chronic bacterial hyper-sensitivity dermatitis is shown.
(a) How would you describe this lesion?
(b) How do the early lesions in this disease appear?
(c) What is the proposed pathomechanism for this disorder in the dog?

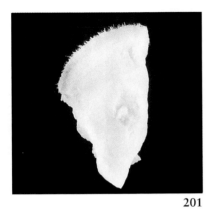

201

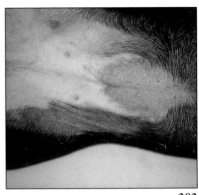

202

201 A 3-year-old domestic short-haired cat developed a firm swelling in the interscapular area. The mass is approximately 3 cm in diameter and is located within the dermis and subcutis, but does not involve the scapular bones. The owners report that the mass was not present three months previously, when the cat was presented to the veterinarian for routine physical examination and vaccination. A cross-section of the mass is shown.
(a) What is the diagnosis?
(b) What is the cause of the mass?

202 The 8-month-old mixed Pit Bull terrier shown presented with a 2-week history of ventral erythema and pruritic urticaria. Skin scrapings were negative for mites, and no external parasites were evident. Faecal flotation revealed hookworm and whipworm ova.
(a) Could this patient's dermatitis be related to the intestinal parasites?
(b) How is the diagnosis of intestinal parasite hypersensitivity made?
(c) What other clinical presentations have been reported in association with intestinal parasite hypersensitivity in the dog?

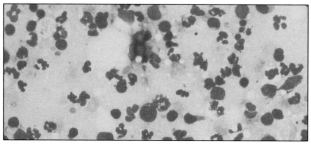

203

203 A 5-year-old Labrador retriever is presented for evaluation of lethargy, weight loss and numerous draining lesions on the extremities. Cytologic examination of the exudate reveals the organisms shown above.
(a) What is the organism?
(b) What further evaluation of the patient is indicated?
(c) Is this a zoonotic disease?

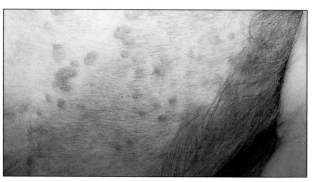

204

204 A few of the many lesions found on physical examination of this 9-year-old neutered male Shetland sheepdog are shown. The owner noted that the lesions would regress spontaneously and that other lesions would appear at adjacent or distant sites.
(a) What is the diagnosis?
(b) Are there any known breed predilections?

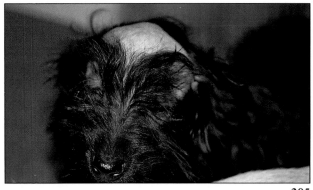

205

205 This 11-week-old male mixed Poodle puppy was born with an obvious lack of hair on his head and entire ventrum. The histopathologic diagnosis (which certainly is consistent with the patient's history) is congenital alopecia/congenital hypotrichosis.
(a) How common is this skin abnormality in the dog?
(b) At what age is the disease evident?
(c) Is there any sex predilection?
(d) Are there any breed predilections?

206 This 4-year-old male black American Cocker spaniel presented with a history of dramatic, rapid, truncal hair loss. The hair loss started several days after he received his yearly vaccinations.
(a) What is the diagnosis?
(b) How is the diagnosis made?
(c) What is the treatment?
(d) Do these patients recover completely?

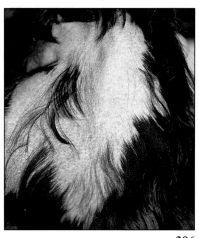

206

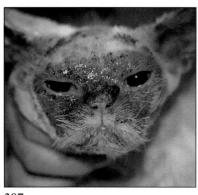

207

207 This 5-year-old female spayed blue-point Siamese cat presented with a several-week history of an ulcerative dermatosis involving mainly the face, ear pinnae and oral mucosa. Many of the footpads were sloughing and the patient was quite painful.
(a) What are the three most important diagnostic tests for this patient?
(b) What is the diagnosis?
(c) List several non-cutaneous signs/abnormalities which may also be present.

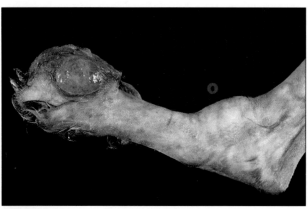

208

208 The masses present on the metatarsal region of a 9-year-old female Briard are shown. This mass is a recurrence of a mass removed from the same site 2 months previously.
(a) What is the most likely diagnosis?
(b) What is the best treatment for this patient?
(c) Where would you expect to find metastasis?

209 The clinical (**A**) and cross-section (**B**) of a single mass arising on the thorax of a 9-year-old miniature Schnauzer are shown. The owner noticed the mass approximately three months prior to presentation. Cytologic examination of an aspirate from the mass revealed epithelial cells, with fairly extensive cytoplasm, and 'ghost-like' nuclei.
(a) What are the two primary differential diagnoses?
(b) Discuss the differences between the two differentials.

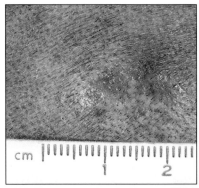

209A

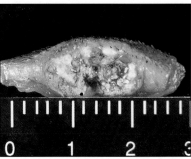

209B

210 The lateral thoracic area of a 9-year-old mixed-breed dog is pictured. The patient developed skin lesions over the past four months. He had no prior history of skin disease. The referring veterinarian prescribed an appropriate course of antibiotic therapy, but the lesions continued to spread and worsen in severity. The patient is non-pruritic. Close examination of the lesions reveals papules, crusts, and occasional pustules. Skin scrapings were negative and a fungal culture revealed no significant growth. Bloodwork was normal, except for an elevated white blood cell count.
(a) What is a major differential diagnosis in this case?
(b) How would you confirm the diagnosis?
(c) What is the treatment?

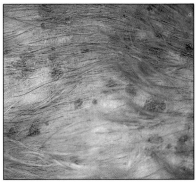

210

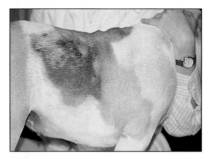

211

211 This 4-year-old female spayed English bulldog has a 2-year history of a waxing and waning hair loss on her lateral thoracic areas. The underlying skin is hyperpigmented. All endocrine tests were within normal limits.
(a) What is the diagnosis?
(b) How is the diagnosis made?
(c) What is the treatment?
(d) What other breeds show a very similar waxing and waning (seasonal?) flank alopecia?

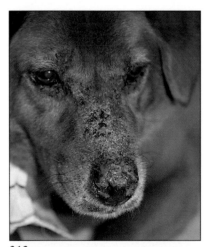

212

212 An 8-year-old neutered male mixed-breed dog is presented with depigmentation and ulceration of the nose as well as crusting of the bridge of the nose and extending, to a lesser degree, to the periocular areas. The patient is non-pruritic, not in pain and feels well.
(a) What are your differential diagnoses?
(b) What is the diagnosis?
(c) What diagnostic tests would you use to confirm your diagnosis?

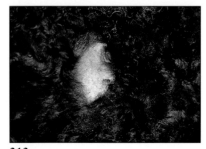

213

213 This 6-year-old male neutered Miniature Poodle presented with an area of total alopecia over the right shoulder. The owner reported that the hair loss was noticed 6 – 8 weeks after the patient received his yearly vaccinations.
(a) What is the diagnosis?
(b) How is the diagnosis made?
(c) What is the treatment?

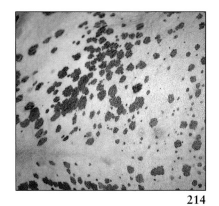

214

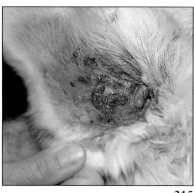

215

214 This 11-year-old mixed Alaskan malamute presented with a several-month history of 'abnormal black spots on the belly'. Physical examination revealed hundreds of pigmented macules on the abdomen. The rest of the physical examination was within normal limits, except for a very brittle hair coat and no palpable testes. On further questioning, the owners reported that they adopted the dog at 2 years of age from a friend and assumed that the dog had been neutered.
(a) What is your number one cause for the patient's abnormal pigmentation?
(b) How would your confirm this diagnosis?

215 This 4-year-old white German shepherd dog has 2.5-year history of recurrent otitis externa. The otitis responds temporarily to combinations of systemic cortico-steroids and antibiotics.
(a) List the five most common differentials for recurrent otitis externa in a 4-year-old dog.
(b) What is the treatment?

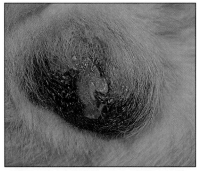

216 This 7-year-old male intact mixed-breed German shepherd dog presented with scrotal dermatitis which was noticed by the owners a few days prior to presentation. Physical examination revealed no other skin or mucocutaneous abnormalities.

(a) What are the two major causes of scrotal ulceration in the canine?

(b) What is the treatment?

216

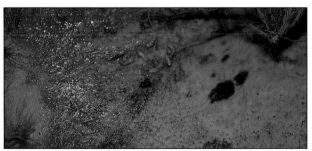

217

217 This 11-month-old mixed-breed dog was presented for a second opinion. The patient was being treated for generalised demodicosis with weekly amitraz dips (appropriately); however, the owner was quite concerned because, after initial improvement, the skin disease seemed to worsen after the seventh dip. The patient was kept outside during the day in a very clean environment, but the temperatures had been quite warm. Physical examination revealed generalised, partial alopecia, varying degrees of erythema, ulceration and secondary bacterial skin infection. The ulcerated abdomen of this patient is shown. On very close observation, several whitish-yellow/grey organisms, approximately one centimetre in diameter, were found on the ulcerated abdominal lesions.

(a) What are these organisms?

(b) What is the treatment?

(c) What precautionary steps should be taken?

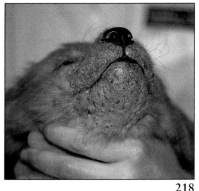

218

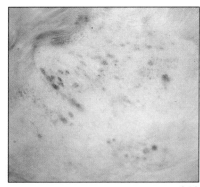

219

218 This 10-week-old Golden retriever puppy presented with a 2-week history of skin disease, which started with swelling of the muzzle, periocular areas, and ear pinnae. The swelling progressed to alopecia and erythema, and the pup developed papules on the abdomen. Physical examination revealed a 'depressed' puppy with enlarged submandibular and inguinal lymph nodes. The pup also had a slight fever.
(a)   What is the diagnosis?
(b)   What is the aetiology of this disease?
(c)   What is the treatment?

219 This 13-year-old Siamese cat had been receiving monthly gold salt injections for three years to control his pemphigus foliaceous. The patient was free of skin lesions until several days prior to re-presentation. The owner noticed that 'new' lesions were developing on the abdomen. Physical examination revealed an overweight, depressed cat, with a slightly subnormal temperature. Numerous petechia and ecchymoses were found on the entire body, but were most evident on the gums and abdomen. An 'in-house' hematocrit was 27%.
(a)   What is happening with this patient?
(b)   How would you manage him?

220 Name the one clinical sign or laboratory abnormality listed below which does not occur in hypothyroid dogs:
(a) Lethargy.
(b) Weight gain.
(c) Hyperexcitability.
(d) Hypercholesterolemia.
(e) Normochromic, nonmycotic anaemia.
(f) Heat seeking.

221 Pancytopenia is an occasional finding in which of the following canine endocrinopathies?
(a) Sertoli cell tumour.
(b) Hyperadrenocorticism.
(c) Hypothyroidism.
(d) Growth hormone-'responsive' dermatosis.

222 In cases of canine oral eosinophilic granuloma:
(a) How is the diagnosis made?
(b) What diseases would you include in your differential diagnoses?
(c) How is this disorder treated?

223 Of the following dermatologic disorders, which is the Chinese Shar pei not predisposed to?
(a) Idiopathic mucinosis.
(b) Bacterial folliculitis.
(c) Allergic inhalant disease (atopy).
(d) Demodicosis (generalised).
(e) Hypothyroidism.
(f) Fold dermatitis.
(g) Seborrhoeic disorders.

224 Regarding the use of antihistamines in the treatment of allergic inhalant disease (atopy) in the canine patient, which of the following is/are not true?
(a) One of the side effects of antihistamines in the canine patient is drowsiness.
(b) Antihistamines bind to both H1 and H2 receptors and exert their effects in this manner.

(c) Antihistamines may directly inhibit or stimulate mast cell secretion.

(d) Antihistamines may change the number, activity or both of helper or suppressor T-lymphocytes.

(e) Antihistamines may activate eosinophils.

225 Which of the following list of substances have been reported as causes of naturally occurring, 'allergic contact dermatitis' in the dog and the cat? Grass resins, tree pollens, weed pollens, poison ivy, poison oak, wandering Jew, neomycin, tetracaine, tar shampoos, petrolatum, lanolin, wool, nylon, synthetics, household polishes.

226 Only about 10% of canine hyperadrenocorticoid patients are pruritic. In order for a 'Cushing's' patient to be pruritic, one of several clinical conditions must be present. List at least two of these.

227 There are five canine skin tumours that are morphologically classified as 'round cell' tumours. Please list them.

228 Regarding the use of fatty acid supplements as anti-inflammatory agents in the treatment of canine allergic inhalant disease (atopy), which of the following statements are true?

(a) Polyunsaturated fatty acids are necessary for caloric energy and the formation and maintenance of the fluidity and function of cell membranes.

(b) The oxidative metabolism of certain fatty acids results in the formation of eicosanoids, which include the prostaglandins and leucotrienes.

(c) Eicosapentanoic acid (EPA), found in marine liquids, is metabolized to the three-series of eicosanoids, which is believed to be anti-inflammatory.

(d) Linoleic, linolenic and arachadonic acids are essential fatty acids. The dog can synthesise both arachadonic and linolenic acids from linoleic acid.

(e) In general, reports using fatty acids as therapy in canines with allergic inhalant disease (atopy) have shown a decrease in clinical signs and improvement of the hair coat, but certainly not (in most cases) the cessation of pruritus.

229 Please match the following canine epithelial neoplasms with the breed of dog, based upon the known/reported breed predilections for these neoplasms in canine skin.

(a) Hepatoid gland adenoma.   ( ) Basset hound.
(b) Subungual squamous cell carcinoma.   ( ) Siberian husky.
(c) Intracutaneous cornifying epithelioma.   ( ) Kerry Blue terrier.
(d) Sebaceous adenoma.   ( ) giant Schnauzer.
(e) Trichoepithelioma.   ( ) Norwegian elkhound.
(f) Pilomatrixoma.   ( ) American Cocker spaniel.

230 The following clinical cutaneous signs are frequently seen in canine patients with hyperadrenocorticism (Cushing's disease). Which of these signs is the most specific for this disease?
(a) Truncal alopecia.
(b) Hyperpigmentation.
(c) Calcinosis cutis.
(d) Seborrhoeic abnormalities.
(e) Recurrent pyoderma.

231 Hepatoid gland tumours (also referred to as perianal gland or circumanal gland tumours), occur primarily in the perianal region of the dog. In what other canine body sites may they also arise?

232 Please answer the following questions regarding hormonal hypersensitivity in the dog and the dermatologic changes it causes.
(a) Is this disease seen more frequently in male dogs or in female dogs?
(b) What type of hypersensitivity reaction is thought to be responsible for this disorder?
(c) How is this disorder treated?

233 An 8-year-old female spayed Irish setter is presented with a small, non-pigmented mass on the right upper eyelid. The owners noticed the mass 2 – 3 months prior to presentation. The lesion does not bother the dog.
(a) What is the most common differential diagnosis?
(b) What are the two names that are used to describe the gland of origin of the mass?
(c) Is this a modified apocrine, eccrine or sebaceous gland?

234 List four systemic signs that may be found in association with canine mast cell tumours. Please explain why each of these signs occurs.

235 Please answer the following questions regarding dermoid sinuses (cysts) in the canine.
(a) Which breed of dog is highly predisposed to the development of this disorder?
(b) In the predisposed breed, what is the mode of inheritance?
(c) At what age are the lesions usually noticed?
(d) Where are the lesions usually located?
(e) Describe what these sinuses (cysts) actually are.

236 Regarding squamous cell carcinoma, please answer the following questions:
(a) What is the aetiology of squamous cell carcinoma in domestic animals and man?
(b) What factors are of importance in determining the location on the body where these tumours are most likely to arise?
(c) In what anatomical location are squamous cell carcinomas most frequently found in:
1 The feline patient? 2 The canine patient?

237 Match the following mesenchymal neoplasms and the canine breed, based upon the predilection of the breed for development of these neoplasms:
(a) Cutaneous liposarcoma. ( ) Boxer.
(b) Cutaneous hemangioma. ( ) Scottish terrier.
(c) Cutaneous hemangiosarcoma. ( ) American Cocker spaniel.
(d) Cutaneous histiocytoma. ( ) Shetland sheepdog.
(e) Cutaneous mast cell tumour. ( ) German shepherd dog.
(f) Cutaneous plasmacytoma. ( ) Airedale terrier.

238 Acute moist dermatitis ('hot spots', pyotraumatic dermatitis) is a common presenting sign in canine veterinary dermatology. Please list at least five predisposing factors for this disease.

239 A 5-year-old male intact miniature Schnauzer has a 1-year history of alopecia of the dorsal trunk with papules and encrusted nodules. The owner reports that pruritus is minimal. Skin scrapings and a fungal culture are negative. There is no evidence of fleas, and the owner uses routine pet and environmental flea control.

(a) What is your tentative diagnosis?

(b) How would you confirm this diagnosis?

(c) What is the treatment?

240 A young male neutered cat presented with a pruritic papulo-crustous eruption involving the dorsal lumbo-sacral area and neck. There was obvious self-induced alopecia. A small amount of flea excreta was found using a flea comb. The owners reported that the skin condition seemed to be more severe in the warmer months.

(a) What is the name given to this cutaneous reaction in the feline?

(b) What are the underlying aetiologies for this skin reaction pattern in the cat?

(c) What diagnostic tests could be useful in making the diagnosis of flea allergy dermatitis in this patient?

241 A 3-year-old female spayed Chow Chow has a 2-year history of non-pruritic alopecia. She was spayed at 9 months of age. Skin scrapings and a fungal culture were negative. A complete blood count and chemistry profile, as well as thyroid and adrenal function tests, were within normal limits. A skin biopsy was non-diagnostic, but suggestive of an endocrine imbalance.

(a) What are your two major differentials in this case?

(b) How would you arrive at your diagnosis?

(c) What is the therapy?

(d) What precautions should be taken with the therapy?

242 A 3-year-old neutered male Airedale terrier has a 1-year history of non-pruritic, bilaterally symmetric alopecia of the flank areas. The owners report that the the alopecic areas vary in size slightly throughout the year, but never resolve. Adrenal and thyroid function tests were within normal limits. Skin scrapings and a fungal culture were negative.

(a) What is your most likely diagnosis?

(b) How is this diagnosis made?

(c) What is the appropriate treatment?

243 A young male intact Scottish terrier had a history of cephalosporin antibiotic administration approximately 10 days prior to presentation for a

urinary tract infection. The patient presented with severe, focal areas of cutaneous necrosis and ulceration. Most of the lesions involved the trunk and the abdomen.
(a) What is the probable diagnosis?
(b) When this diagnosis is made, what is the most common route of administration of the offending agent?
(c) How is the diagnosis made?
(d) What is the treatment?

244 A 12-year-old intact male mixed-breed dog presented with physical changes that are typically associated with 'male feminising syndrome'.
(a) List the classic changes.
(b) What is the most important part of the physical examination, other than very careful cutaneous examination?
(c) What is the presumed cause of the physical/cutaneous changes?

245 A 14-year-old female spayed Airedale terrier was presented with numerous cutaneous masses. The masses involved mainly the trunk, but a few were present on the face and legs. The lesions were non-painful and non-pruritic. A previous biopsy revealed that the masses were 'not cancerous' and involved the sebaceous glands.
(a) What is your major differential diagnosis?
(b) What is the clinical significance of these lesions and their biologic behaviour?

246 Regarding sarcoptic mange (scabies) in canine patients in a kennel situation, please answer the following questions:
(a) What are the two 'best' tests to confirm a diagnosis of canine sarcoptic mange?
(b) What treatment steps would you initiate?

247 A 9-year-old male German shepherd dog was purchased at 2 years of age. When the pet was purchased, he was taken to the veterinarian for a complete physical examination and vaccinations. Since no testicles were palpable, it was assumed that he was neutered. At approximately 8 years of age, the owners noticed increased pigment in the skin involving the abdomen and medial thighs. Soon after, the dog's nipples began to enlarge. The patient

was not pruritic. He was presented to his veterinarian for evaluation of this condition.
(a) What is the most likely diagnosis?
(b) How can you confirm this?
(c) What is the treatment?

248 A 4-year-old neutered male domestic short-haired cat presented with a history of recurring hair loss. The pattern consistently involved the ventro-lateral thoraco-lumbar areas as well as the rear legs and abdomen. The owners did not notice excessive grooming of these areas or any evidence that the hair loss was 'self-induced'.
(a) How would you determine whether or not the hair loss was self-induced or spontaneous?
(b) What are the three major causes of self-induced hair loss in the feline?
(c) This condition is very commonly misdiagnosed. What is the most common misdiagnosis?

249 A 6-month-old male intact mixed-breed puppy had a 5-week history of alopecia, erythema and crusting around the eyes, on the muzzle and on various pressure points. The owners reported that the dog was not pruritic. They also reported that he appeared to have a low energy level. His diet consisted of 'whichever dog food was the cheapest', and he was not given dietary supplements of any kind. Skin scrapings were negative for demodectic mites, and a fungal culture revealed no significant growth.
(a) What is your tentative diagnosis?
(b) How would you confirm this?
(c) What is the treatment?

250 An obese 11-year-old female dog is presented with a 1 – 2-year history of numerous subcutaneous masses. The masses are round-to-oval, smooth, soft, circumscribed and vary in diameter from 2 – 8 cm.
(a) What is the most likely diagnosis?
(b) What is the significance of these tumours?

ANSWERS

1 (a) Allergic inhalant disease (atopy).
(b) Subcutaneous injections of methyl-prednisolone acetate may be used safely in most feline patients at a dosage of 2 mg per pound of body weight, not to be used more frequently than every 3 months. If more frequent use of corticosteroids is needed, intradermal allergy testing and hyposensitization are recommended.
(c) Flea bite hypersensitivity, food hypersensitivity, ear mites (*Otodectes cynotis*), *Cheyletiella* infestation and notoedric mange.

2 (a) The six major differential diagnoses for non-pruritic crusts around the eyes are:
1 Bacterial pyoderma. 2 Dermatophytosis. 3 Demodicosis. 4 Pemphigus foliaceous.
5 Superficial necrolytic dermatitis (hepatocutaneous syndrome). 6 Zinc-responsive dermatosis.
(b) A skin biopsy would be the most advantageous diagnostic test to run at this point, as it will in most cases distinguish between a folliculitis (differential diagnoses 1 – 3) and the other diseases listed. It is important not to perform any preparation of the skin prior to biopsy, as this will alter or destroy the stratum corneum, wherein may lie the diagnosis. The histology of the skin from this dog had extensive parakeratosis (retained nuclei in the stratum corneum), with a slightly acanthotic epidermis, consistent with zinc-responsive dermatosis.

3 (a) Castration-responsive dermatosis. The distribution of the hair coat changes and lack of pruritus suggest an endocrinopathy. The biopsy confirms this. The early age of onset eliminates other endocrine diseases (hypothyroidism, hyperadrenocorticism).
(b) Although some of the dogs may exhibit abnormalities on serum sex hormone evaluation, the only confirmation of this disease is to neuter the dog. The hair coat generally returns to normal within 4 months after surgery.

4 (a) Frostbite, fly strike and vasculitis.
(b) Coomb's test at 4° C and autoagglutination of whole blood in EDTA on a slide at temperatures below 30° C.

5 (a) Alopecia areata.
(b) Corticosteroids have been used, but their benefit is questionable.
(c) Some dogs will spontaneously regrow hair in 6 months to several years.

6 (a) Canine allergic inhalant disease (atopy).
(b) Breeds of dogs that are genetically predisposed to this disease include Labrador retrievers, Golden retrievers, German shepherd dogs, Chinese Shar peis, American Cocker spaniels, Shih tzus, and West Highland White terriers. However, any breed, including mixed breeds, are often affected
(c) Most patients develop signs between 4 months and 4 years of age.
(d) Females appear to be predisposed.
(e) Canine atopy has been classified as a Type I hypersensitivity reaction. The antibody involved is IgE. IgGd subclass antibodies are thought to be involved in the hypersensitivity reaction in some patients.

7 (a) Demodicosis, bacterial folliculitis and dermatophyte infection.
(b) Many deep skin scrapings should be performed to check for *Demodex* mites. It is useful to squeeze the skin prior to scraping, as this helps to force the mites from the hair follicles or sebaceous gland.
— Cytologic examination of material taken from the lesions may be helpful in demonstrating cocci which would be present in large numbers in cases of bacterial folliculitis.
— A Wood's lamp would show positive fluorescence in most cases of *Microsporum canis*.
— A dermatophye culture is the most accurate diagnostic test for canine and feline ringworm

(dermatophyte) infections. The area to be cultured should be gently wiped with alcohol and hairs plucked from the peripheral area of the lesion and placed on the appropriate dermatophyte test media. Patients with dermatophyte infections have positive cultures in 4 – 14 days. The culture growth should be stained and examined microscopically to determine the causative agent, which is especially important in zoonotic infections.

Note: The patient shown has a dermatophyte infection caused by *Microsporum canis*.

8 (a) This disease is seen most commonly in young dogs with breed predilection for those canines with a heavy, dense pelage, such as the Golden retriever, Labrador retriever, collie, German shepherd dog and St. Bernard. There is no sex predilection noted for this disease. The incidence increases in hot and humid weather.

(b) The majority of cases of acute moist dermatitis are due to flea bite allergy. Other underlying disorders include various allergic skin diseases (food, inhalants), other ectoparasites, anal sac inflammation, otitis externa, foreign bodies in the coat, irritant substances (shampoos and dips), dirty and unkempt coats, psychoses, fatty acid deficiencies and painful musculoskeletal disorders.

(c) A recent study has examined areas of acute moist dermatitis histopathologically and demonstrated that they could be classified into two groups. In one group the lesions did not have a significant bacterial component. They were superficial, ulcerative, inflammatory processes. The second group also had superficial ulceration, but also deep suppurative and necrotizing folliculitis and occasional furunculosis. Clinically, this type of lesion is thickened, plaque-like, and surrounded by 'satellite' papules and pustules. The second presentation is best treated with systemic antibiotics.

9 (a) No.

(b) Solitary.

(c) 1 – 5 cm.

(d) No. Most patients are late middle age or older.

10 (a) Idiopathic flank alopecia/follicular dysplasia.

(b) Diagnosis is made on the basis of the history revealing a cyclical pattern of recurring and resolving alopecia, physical examination showing that the lesions are typically limited to the flank areas, and ruling out endocrine alopecias such as hypothyroidism and hyperadrenocorticism. Biopsies for histopathologic examination reveal keratin-filled, distorted hair follicles with undulated outline, suggestive of follicular dysplasias. The follicular dysplasias include a number of alopecic diseases which clinically look like endocrine imbalances. Many breeds may be affected, but those predisposed include Boxers, English bulldogs, French bulldogs, Airedale terriers and miniature Schnauzers.

11 (a) Yes; Samoyeds, Akitas and Chow Chows.

(b) No.

(c) Vitiligo (loss of skin pigment) and leucotrichia (loss of hair pigment).

(d) The cutaneous disease usually has only cosmetic significance. The granulomatous uveitis may lead to blindness.

12 (a) Less than 4 years old.

(b) Usually solitary, but may be multiple.

(c) Legs, face and scrotum.

13 (a) Pemphigus vulgaris, systemic lupus erythematosus, severe erythema multiforme, toxic epidermal necrolysis and chemical burn.

(b) The histopathologic diagnosis is toxic epidermal necrolysis.

(c) Antibiotics and vaccinations.
(d) Uncommon to rare.

14 (a) Frostbite, fly strike, septic vasculitis, systemic lupus erythematosus, cold agglutinin disease and immune-mediated vasculitis.
(b) Wedge skin biopsies for histopathologic examination. (The diagnosis is immune-mediated vasculitis.)

15 (a) Tail fold, lip fold, vulvar fold and body fold.
(b) Facial fold dermatitis is seen in brachycephalic breeds, especially Pekingese, English bulldogs and Pugs. Tail fold dermatitis results from pressure of 'corkscrew' tails on the skin of the perineum and is seen most frequently in English bulldogs, Pugs, and Boston terriers. Lip fold dermatitis is prevalent in dogs with a large lip flap, such as spaniels and St. Bernards, especially as the dog starts to develop dental tartar. Vulvar fold dermatitis is common in obese older females that have infantile vulvas as a result of spaying at a young age. Body fold dermatitis is seen in obese individuals, the Chinese Shar pei and some English bulldogs.
(c) Medical treatment may be palliative in many of these cases, but surgical correction of the anatomic defect and elimination of the fold is the only permanent treatment. Drying solutions such as Domboro's (aluminium acetate), followed by a topical cream containing antibiotics/corticosteroids or anti-yeast medication, should be used, based on epidermal cytology from the surface of the lesion.

16 (a) Cutaneous syndromes associated with feline atopy include:
1 Facial pruritus, with or without lesions. 2 Pruritic ears, with or without lesions.
3 A widespread pruritic papulocrustous dermatitis ('miliary dermatitis'). 4 Indolent ulcer, eosinophilic plaque or eosinophilic granuloma. 5 Symmetric alopecia. 6 Generalised pruritus, with or without lesions.
(b) In cats, 75% of affected animals initially manifest clinical signs between 6 months and 2 years old. No breed or sex predilections have been reported for feline atopy.
(c) Definitive laboratory documentation, including the characterisation of the reaginic antibody in the cat (IgE? IgG) has not been accomplished. One group has reported isolation of feline IgE for use in an *in vitro* allergy test.

17 (a) Dermatophytosis caused by *Microsporum canis*.
(b) The most important treatment goals are to limit spread of the disease to other susceptible animals, minimise the spread of the contagion and attempt to hasten recovery of the affected animal with appropriate therapy. In order to limit the spread of the disease to other animals, the cat should be quarantined in the owner's home. All animals in contact with the affected cat should be treated and also quarantined. The most effective method of minimising the spread of this infectious disease is to clip the kitten's hair coat to remove the infected hairs. This material should be burned. In addition, the owner should thoroughly clean and disinfect the house with common household bleach. Dermatophytosis is often a self-limiting disease if re-exposure does not occur, and if left untreated this kitten's infection may eventually resolve. However, dermatophytosis is a contagious and zoonotic disease and, therefore, treatment is warranted. Topical, whole body treatment with an appropriate antifungal agent (e.g. lime sulphur, chlorhexidine, Dermazole®) is required every 5-7 days for a minimum of six weeks. Systemic antifungal agents may be added to the treatment regimen if the infection does not respond to topical therapy alone.

18 (a) Multiple ceruminous cysts.
(b) They occur due to blockage of the duct of the ceruminous gland with retention of the secretion of the glands, which has a black-brown colour when it becomes inspissated.

19 (a) Canine tail gland hyperplasia.
(b) Confirmation is via skin biopsy, which in this case shows sebaceous and perianal gland hyperplasia.
(c) Treatment involves determining the presence of an underlying disorder, if any, including testicular neoplasia and/or generalised seborrhoea. In a dog such as this, with no obvious testicular abnormalities and no generalised seborrhoea, castration may prove beneficial, with remission of clinical signs within 2 months. (This is because the tail glands are stimulated by testosterone.) Antiseborrhoeic shampoos may be of palliative benefit.
Note: The editor comments that a significant number of canine patients with tail gland hyperplasia are hypothyroid.

20 (a) Usually a secondary response of the skin to an underlying disease.
(b) Food allergy, allergic inhalant disease (atopy), hypothyroidism, sex hormone 'imbalances', demodicosis and hereditary sebaceous gland abnormalities.

21 (a) Sebaceous adenitis. Another possible diagnosis would be castration-responsive dermatosis, but that disease rarely causes the extensive alopecia seen in this patient.
(b) Confirmation is via skin biopsy, which in early lesions reveals a pyogranulomatous to granulomatous infiltrate involving the sebaceous gland. In the late stages of the disease, all inflammation may have resolved following destruction of the sebaceous glands, showing a complete absence of these glands on biopsy.
(c) A number of different treatments are possible. Mildly affected dogs may benefit from antiseborrhoeic shampoos. Spraying the dog with a 50:50 mix of water and propylene glycol on a twice a day basis is very effective both in reducing the amount of scale and in promoting hair-growth, particularly in the long-haired breeds. Utilising essential fatty acid supplements, often at twice their recommended dosage, may benefit some dogs (diarrhoea may be a side-effect). Use of the retinoid drugs, isotretinoin or etretinate, at a dosage of 1 mg/kg per day will help promote hair-regrowth, particularly in Viszlas. (The use of these drugs must be carefully monitored via frequent CBCs and chemistry profiles.)

22 (a) Hock callous with secondary bacterial infection.
(b) Pressure point callouses are more prominent in patients exposed to hard surfaces such as cement or linoleum. They are also accentuated in hypothyroid dogs as well as patients with underlying internal disorders such as hypothyroidism and Cushing's disease. (Intense pruritus of the elbows and hocks with associated excoriations and callous formation is seen in patients with sarcoptic mange.)

23 (a) 1 Plaque stage—the disease presents with single or multiple erythematous plaques.
2 Tumour stage—solitary or, more commonly, multiple, intradermal and/or subcutaneous masses. 3 Erythematous stage—erythematous lesions of varying size with alopecia and excessive white adherent scale formation.
(b) Erythematous stage.

24 (a) Oestrogen-responsive dermatosis (hypo-oestrogenism, ovarian imbalance type II).
(b) Other endocrinopathies would be unlikely to manifest themselves at such an early age; lack of response to thyroid hormone further rules out this differential diagnosis. Hair regrowth with administration of oral oestrogen (1 mg, three times a week for 6 weeks, then as needed) will confirm the diagnosis. Bone marrow suppression may be a side effect of oestrogen therapy.

25 (a) The most likely diagnosis is atypical mycobacterial infection. The two most common mycobacterial organisms responsible for this infection in the cat are *Mycobacterium fortuitum* and *Mycobacterium chelonei.*

(b)   The lesions are most commonly found on the caudal abdomen and dorsally over the lower back and pelvic areas. They are thought to occur after a traumatic event such as a cat fight, and seem most able to establish infection when inoculation of the organisms occurs into the subcutaneous tissues.

(c)   The course of infection is long and the prognosis is guarded. Lesions may regress spontaneously after several months, with or without treatment. The most successful therapy is wide surgical excision, debridement, systemic antibiotics and local treatment. If possible, sensitivity testing should be carried out. Currently, enrofloxacin is the initial antibiotic of choice. Laboratory antibiotic sensitivity to kanamycin, gentamicin and amikacin, has been reasonably reliable, with less dependable sensitivity to erythromycin, chloramphenicol, tetracycline and polymyxin.

26   (a)   Feline eosinophilic plaque.

(b)   Differential diagnoses include infectious granulomas (bacterial, fungal) and neoplasia (mast cell tumour, lymphosarcoma); many, if not all, cases of feline eosinophilic plaque are associated with underlying hypersensitivity responses such as flea bite hypersensitivity, atopy or food hypersensitivity.

(c)   The other area of predilection for eosinophilic plaque is the abdomen.

27   (a)   The differential diagnoses for generalised mucocutaneous ulceration include systemic lupus erythematosus (SLE), pemphigus vulgaris (PV), bullous pemphigoid (BP), drug reaction and mucocutaneous candidiasis.

(b)   The autoimmune skin diseases (SLE, PV, BP) would be differentiated from each other by physical examination (SLE would involve more than one body system), histopathological examination of a skin biopsy specimen and specialised laboratory tests (antinuclear antibody testing). Drug reactions can mimic almost any skin disease. However, the history of the administration of a drug and improvement of clinical signs upon withdrawal of the drug are very suggestive of a drug reaction/eruption. Mucocutaneous candidiasis can be diagnosed via skin biopsy, culture, or more commonly by cytologic examination of the exudate from the affected areas. Tentative diagnosis of candidiasis should be confirmed via culture.

(c)   The organism is *Candida* spp. Mucocutaneous candidiasis is a rare disease that occurs in animals with predisposing diseases or factors (excessive moisture, debilitation, and lowered host resistance).

(d)   Clinical management of these patients requires identification of the underlying/predisposing cause, if possible. Excessive moisture must be avoided. Hair in the affected areas should be clipped and the lesions washed with a mild cleansing shampoo/solution. Topical nystatin, clotrimazole or miconazole are effective. In severe cases, ketoconazole may be effective.

28   (a)   Feline hyperadrenocorticism (Cushing's disease). Cats' skin collagen may alter with this disease, causing the skin to become friable (just as dogs' collagen may alter with hyper-adrenocorticism, causing it to attract mineralisation: calcinosis cutis).

(b)   Confirmation may be by ACTH stimulation or dexamethasone-suppression tests. However, the regimens for these tests have not yet been standardised in a large series of cats with this disease; in addition, they may not distinguish between pituitary-dependent hyperadrenocorticism and a functional adrenal tumour. Alternative methods of diagnosis are ultrasounding the abdomen (looking for unilateral or bilateral adrenal enlargement) and exploratory surgery.

(c)   Prognosis is generally poor when the skin has become friable. Typically, the diabetes mellitus in these cats is difficult to control. Some success has been reported in isolated cases with ketoconazole treatment, and also with bilateral adrenalectomy (and subsequent management of the patient as a hypoadrenocorticism case).

29 (a) Ovariohysterectomy-responsive dermatosis, hyperoestrogenism, ovarian imbalance type I. Other endocrinopathies such as hypothyroidism and hyperadrenocorticism usually have truncal hair coat changes without the perianal and perivulvar changes seen in this patient.
(b) Thyroid and adrenal function tests will rule out abnormalities in these organs. Elevated serum oestrogen (and occasionally progesterone) values are seen in some dogs, however normal sex hormone serum levels are often present in involved patients. The only absolute (but obviously irreversible) treatment is ovariohysterectomy. Cystic ovaries are frequently found upon examination of the reproductive tract. The hair coat and skin generally return to normal within 2 – 6 months after ovariohysterectomy.

30 (a) Systemic lupus erythematosus.
(b) Many cases respond to non-corticosteroid drugs such as tetracycline and niacinamide. However, at least 25% of DLE patients have severe nasal ulceration and erosion requiring potentially unsafe levels of corticosteroids and other immunosuppresive medications.

31 (a) Feline hypothyroidism.
(b) Very rare.
(c) L-thyroxine at a dosage of 0.1 mg per 4.5 kg of body weight once or twice daily.

32 Vaccination of the dog with an autologous papilloma virus vaccine to prevent the dog from developing oral papillomatosis while on a drug trail. Some dogs will develop a squamous cell carcinoma at the vaccination site. The latency period varies from 1 – 3 years. Papillomavirus can be demonstrated within the tumour by immunohistochemical methods.

33 (a) The most likely diagnosis is nocardiosis.
(b) Diagnosis is made by direct smear, aerobic culture and biopsy. Histopathology reveals nodular-to-diffuse dermatitis or panniculitis or both, with or without tissue grains.
(c) Clinical management includes surgical drainage of infected tissues and antibacterial therapy. Large doses of penicillin and a sulphonamide, or sulphadiazine by itself, are helpful. Equal parts of sulphadiazine and trimethoprim are probably best. The course of treatment usually continues for several months and should not stop until 4 weeks after clinical remission.

34 (a) Flea bite hypersensitivity (flea allergy dermatitis).
(b) In addition to immediate reactivity, animals may go through a period of delayed hypersensitivity to the flea where skin test reactivity would be positive if checked at 48 – 72 hours.
(c) The differential diagnosis for flea allergy dermatitis in the dog would include food hypersensitivity, atopy, drug hypersensitivity, intestinal parasite hypersensitivity, sarcoptic mange, and folliculitis.

35 (a) The working diagnosis is a primary disorder of keratinisation with secondary pruritus and *Malassezia* otitis and dermatitis.
(b) The role of *Malassezia* in skin disease is controversial, however it is becoming apparent that this commensal organism is an opportunistic pathogen that flourishes in skin that is oily, moist, or inflamed. It is uncertain if *Malassezia* can act as a primary pathogen.
(c) In this patient's case, control of proliferation of *Malassezia* is dependent upon minimising the microclimatic skin conditions that favour its growth. Frequent bathing with an antiseborrhoeic shampoo will decrease accumulations of oil. Ketoconazole, chlorhexidine or selenium sulphide shampoos may be beneficial adjuvant therapy in cases of acute exacerbations. Oral ketoconazole can effectively resolve *Malassezia* infections; however, the organism will flourish again if the underlying factors return.

36 (a) Seborrhoea sicca.

(b) Poor nutrition, intestinal parasites, too frequent bathing, hypothyroidism and demodicosis.

37 (a) 1 The stubbly hairs examined under a microscope reveal that they have normal hair bulbs and frayed ends, indicating that the hair loss is self-induced. 2 Finding fleas or flea excreta on the patient using a flea comb. (Cats are such fastidious groomers that evidence of fleas in a flea allergic feline may not be found.) 3 Intradermally injected flea antigen reveals an immediate positive reaction in flea-allergic patients.
(b) Food hypersensitivity and allergic inhalant disease (atopy).
(c) Feline endocrine alopecia, which is extremely rare.

38 (a) There is no classical cutaneous syndrome associated with food hypersensitivity in the dog. It can mimic numerous other dermatologic diseases. A variety of primary and secondary skin lesions are seen in food allergy, including papules, plaques, pustules, wheals, erythema, ulcers, excoriations, scales and crusts.
(b) The diagnosis of food hypersensitivity is made by feeding the animals a hypoallergenic diet for a minimum of 6 – 8 weeks. Hypoallergenic diets must be individualised for each patient, based on careful dietary history. The objectives of the diet are:
1 To feed the animals dietary substances that they are not commonly exposed to; and, 2 To feed the animals a diet that is free of additives (colourings, flavourings, preservatives).
(c) Although classical veterinary dermatologic literature states that food hypersensitivity in the dog is not corticosteroid–responsive, a more recent study showed that greater than 70% of a group of 54 food-allergic dogs showed beneficial response to corticosteroid therapy.
Note: Recently popular serum ELISA and RAST tests for food allergy in the dog and cat are considered by most veterinary dermatologists and allergists to be highly inaccurate, and are not recommended.

39 (a) Sterile nodular panniculitis.
(b) Biopsies for histopathologic examination are the most important tests. Negative bacterial and fungal cultures of the exudate, as well as negative skin scrapings for demodectic mites, are also important.
(c) High dosages of corticosteroids are essential. The starting dose should be close to 1 mg per kg of body weight twice daily, then decreasing as the lesions improve. The editor does not prescribe concurrent antibiotics; however, many dermatologists feel that antibiotics are helpful.

40 (a) Juvenile pyoderma (puppy strangles, puppy cellulitis).
(b) Immunosuppressive doses of corticosteroids.
(c) The pathogenesis is not known, but since this disease responds so dramatically to immunosuppressive doses of corticosteroids, it is believed by some to be an autoimmune/immune-mediated disease, possibly associated with vaccination.

41 (a) Digital hyperkeratosis.
(b) Pemphigus foliaceus, zinc dermatopathy, generic dog food dermatosis, hypothyroidism, lupus erythematosus, American Cocker spaniel seborrhoeic disease and idiopathic sebhorrhoeic or keratinisation disease.

42 (a) No.
(b) Chinese Crested (hairless).
(c) 'Hairless' and powderpuff.

43 (a) Pemphigus foliaceus and pemphigus erythematosus. (The diagnosis is pemphigus erythematosus.)
(b) Skin biopsies for histopathologic examination.
(c) No.

44 (a)   The lesions should first be treated with systemic corticosteroids and antibiotics. Once there is significant improvement, a low-allergen diet should be fed to the cat for 6 – 8 weeks. (The exact diet depends upon the dietary history of the patient. Any foods the patient has previously eaten should not be part of the diet. Two commonly used allergy test diets are lamb and rice, and rabbit and rice.)

(b)   Flea bite hypersensitivity, allergic inhalant disease (atopy), ear mites (*Otodectes cynotis*), notoedric mange and *Cheyletiella* infestation.

45 (a)   Canine cutaneous histiocytoma.

(b)   These tumours are quite benign. A proportion of them will regress spontaneously, but some require surgical excision. Less than 1% will recur at the site of surgical excision.

(c)   The English bulldog, Scottish terrier, Greyhound, Boxer and Boston terrier are all predisposed. These breeds have an odds ratio greater than four and a 95% confidence level greater than two for developing this tumour.

(d)   60% of dogs who develop cutaneous histiocytomas are less than 3 years old.

46 (a)   Superficial pustular dermatitis, puppy pyoderma or impetigo.

(b)   This is a bacterial skin infection caused by a coagulase-positive *Staphylococcus intermedius* organism. It is not contagious. It is often a secondary infection associated with intestinal parasitism, external parasitism, viral infections, an unclean environment or poor nutrition. It may also be seen in apparently very clean, healthy puppies. In these patients, an 'immature immune system' may be the underlying predisposition.

(c)   Treatment includes the elimination of the underlying cause(s), if present and detectable. Secondly, topical antibacterial therapy with antibacterial shampoos such as povidone-iodine, chlorhexidine or benzoyl peroxide. Topical antibiotic creams and ointments may be beneficial. Rarely, systemic antibiotics are indicated.

47 (a)   With corticosteroids.

(b)   The clinical signs are consistent with autoimmune skin disease, specifically pemphigus foliaceus, and corticosteroids are inexpensive.

48 (a)   Apocrine carcinoma.

(b)   Multiple deep skin biopsies submitted for histopathologic examination.

(c)   There is often extensive invasion of the dermal lymphatics by the tumour cells. This produces an occlusion of the lymphatics leading to extensive exudation of a serous fluid onto the skin.

(d)   These tumours are exceedingly malignant and metastasize via lymphatics to the regional lymph nodes and to the lungs.

49 (a)   Bacterial folliculitis caused by *Staphylococcus intermedius*.

(b)   These lesions are epidermal collarettes. They are the endstage of pustular lesions.

(c)   Therapy includes an assessment of possible underlying causes or predisposing diseases which contributed to the development of the bacterial lesions/folliculitis. Possible causes are local trauma such as bruising and/or scratching, poor grooming, underlying seborrhoeic abnormalities, parasites, hormonal imbalances, local irritants (shampoos, flea dips) and allergic dermatitis. Systemic antibiotics are indicated for a minimum of 3 weeks.

50 (a)   Very rare.

(b)   Yes. Other predisposed breeds include the West Highland White terrier, Irish setter, Labrador retriever and collie.

(c)   There is really no treatment that allows severe ichthyotic patients to live a comfortable life.

51 (a)   Growth hormone-responsive alopecia, adult-onset hyposomatotropism. This disease is most commonly reported in Chow Chows, Samoyeds, Keeshonds, Pomeranians and Miniature Poodles. Adult-onset endocrine alopecia in a spayed female Keeshond, in the absence of thyroid and adrenal disease, is most likely growth hormone-responsive alopecia. Oestrogen-responsive alopecia is another differential diagnosis, but this usually involves other areas of the body in addition to the caudal thighs.

(b) Confirmation of this diagnosis involves measuring serum growth hormone levels before and after administration of xylazine (which stimulates growth hormone release at a dosage of 0.3 mg per kg of body weight). This may cause severe hypotension in some patients. Patients with growth hormone-responsive alopecia should have no increase in their serum growth hormone levels one hour after xylazine administration. However, it is very difficult to find laboratories capable of performing valid assays for measuring canine serum growth hormone. Note: Skin biopsies may show abnormal elastin, but this is not always diagnostic. Response to growth hormone injections would be beneficial, but safe, effective growth hormone is quite difficult and expensive to obtain.

52 (a) Peripheral lymphadenopathy, hepatomegaly, splenomegaly, lethargy, anorexia and weight loss.

(b) The Bernese mountain dog is definitely predisposed to systemic histiocytosis, which appears to be a similar disease.

(c) Very poor. Usually death or euthanasia occurs within 6 months of diagnosis.

53 (a) Ear mite infestation (*Otodectes cynotis*).

(b) Microscopic examination of the ear debris may show the mites and/or their eggs. However, since the mite number in some patients is quite low, negative findings on microscopic examination of ear exudate do not rule out a diagnosis of ear mites.

(c) The ears should be thoroughly cleaned and an appropriate miticide instilled. Treatment of the ears should be continued for 6 weeks. In addition, the body of the kitten should be treated with a flea spray or powder for 6 weeks to kill migrating ear mites. Re-infestation of the ears from body mites is common. Finally, ear mites are highly contagious. All animals in contact with the infested kitten should be examined and treated.

54 (a) Callous pyoderma.

(b) Callous formation is the initial response of the skin to trauma. Continuous trauma (such as the elbows of a large or giant breed of dog contacting hard surfaces every time the patient lies down) causes a proliferative skin reaction. Crevices develop in the area, which results in a 'fold' dermatitis. This area of increased moisture and maceration is ideal for a bacterial infection to develop. Continued trauma causes epidermal breakdown, ulceration of pressure points, and fistulas. (The condition is often exacerbated in obese or hypothyroid patients.)

(c) The hocks and the sternum.

(d) Treatment must be directed towards relieving the trauma so that the tissue can heal. T-shirts with padded elbows are quite helpful. The patient should be encouraged to lie on soft surfaces. Antibiotic therapy is usually indicated for 6 – 12 weeks. (Occasionally, surgical excision is used; however, in most cases this procedure worsens the condition.) If the patient is obese, weight loss is essential. If the patient is hypothyroid, this should be immediately corrected.

(e) Long-term prognosis for 'cure' is poor. Obviously, if underlying predisposing factors can be detected and treated (such as irritating sleeping surfaces, obesity and/or hypothyroidism), the prognosis is much better.

55 (a) Ear pinnal margin dermatosis, ear pinnal margin seborrhoeic disease or pinnal pattern alopecia.

(b) These diseases are most commonly seen in short-haired Dachshunds, and the diagnosis is often made on a clinical basis. Confirmation of the diagnosis is possible by skin biopsies submitted for histopathologic examination. However, ear pinnal biopsies are difficult and result in further cosmetic defects.

(c) The hair loss is often permanent. (Some patients have accompanying hypothyroidism, which when treated may allow some hair re-growth.) Seborrhoea of the margin may be helped by the topical application of lubricants and a corticosteroid cream/ointment. (Remember that topical cortisone may further increase hair loss and may delay healing.) In severe cases in which the ear pinnae are fissured and bleeding, the only successful treatment is surgical removal of the distal one-third of the ear pinnae.

56 (a) Deep pyoderma/cellulitis results from extension of a bacterial infection from a hair follicle which ruptures. The infection dissects through the tissues and extends downwards into the deep dermis and subcutaneous tissues.

(b) All the diseases listed as causative disorders for recurrent folliculitis may be precursors for deep pyoderma. In general, an underlying cause is not found, and it is presumed that animals that suffer with recurrent deep pyodermas have specific immune dysfunction, most likely associated with defective cell-mediated immunity, which allows the infections to continue.

(c) Although unusual, bacteremia and septicemia may develop. Any chronic infection may be associated with immune-mediated glomerulonephritis.

57 (a) Feline hyperaesthesia syndrome.

(b) Diagnostics should include testing to rule out kidney disease, radiographs to evaluate the spine in this region, and toxoplasmosis serum titers. If possible, electrodiagnostics to evaluate the muscles and nerves in the area should be performed to look for causative factors. In most of these patients, extensive diagnostic testing fails to reveal an underlying aetiology.

58 (a) Calcinosis circumscripta. The mass consists of islands of material with a chalky consistency, subdivided by connective tissue trabeculae.

(b) The prognosis is excellent following surgical removal. If not removed, the lesion may ossify, producing a firm, intradermal and subcutaneous mass.

(c) These lesions most commonly occur over the joints of young, large-to-giant breed dogs. They are less frequently seen arising on the tongue, and very occasionally involve the ligamentum nuchae.

(d) Tumoural calcinosis.

59 (a) Follicular dysplasia (hypotrichosis) of the Portuguese water dog. Biopsies for histopathologic examination confirm the diagnosis.

(b) Hypothyroidism, hyperadrenocorticism and sex hormone imbalances.

(c) There is no treatment. The hair loss is progressive and permanent.

(d) Siberian husky, Irish water spaniel, Airedale terrier, Curly coated retriever, Boxer, English bulldog, French bulldog, miniature Schnauzer and Dobermann pinscher.

60 (a) Mucocutaneous papillomatosis.

(b) Canine papillomavirus.

(c) Within the oral cavity. Halitosis and excessive salivation are common.

(d) No.

61 (a) Anal sac abscess. A foreign body or a tumour could show similar signs.

(b) Under general anaesthesia, the area should be probed for a foreign body, exudate collected for a bacterial culture and sensitivity, and the remaining exudate flushed out with saline or a diluted chlorhexidine solution. An antibiotic is best prescribed on the basis of the sensitivity results. Systemic antibiotic therapy is required in this case for 4 – 8 weeks. The owners should be instructed to 'hot-pack' the area at least three times daily, for ten minutes each time. If the condition is non-responsive or recurrent, surgical excision of the anal sac(s) is recommended. (In some cases of recurrent anal sac impaction/abscessation, surgery can be prevented by teaching the owners to express the anal sacs every 1 – 2 months.)

62 (a) The cutaneous problems associated with this tick, *Dermacentor variabilis*, imbedding in canine skin are usually minor. There may be erythema at the site of attachment, and if the tick is improperly removed a small granuloma may develop.
(b) Ticks are capable of transmitting a number of 'systemic' diseases which are of far greater significance than the skin irritation. They include: Rocky Mountain spotted fever, St. Louis encephalitis, tularaemia, anaplasmosis, tick paralysis and Lyme's disease.

63 (a) Sebaceous adenitis.
(b) The diagnosis is confirmed by multiple skin biopsies taken for histopathologic examination. Early lesions reveal a pyogranulomatous to granulomatous infiltrate of the sebaceous glands. In the late stages of the disease, all of the inflammation is resolved and there is an absence of sebaceous glands.
(c) Standard Poodles, Viszlas, Akitas and Samoyeds.
(d) 1 Corticosteroids are helpful in some patients. Obviously, long-term therapy may have significant side effects. 2 A 50% solution of propylene glycol sprayed on the skin is helpful in many cases, but may be quite messy. 3 The vitamin A derivatives such as Acutane and Tegison are often beneficial.

64 (a) Superficial necrolytic dermatitis. This disease has also been called the following: hepatic dermatopathy, diabetic dermatopathy, necrolytic migratory erythema and hepatocutaneous syndrome.
(b) Skin biopsies for histopathologic examination reveal layering of the superficial parakeratotic crust, sub-adjacent edema and deep hyperplastic keratinocytes in the epidermis.
(c) Systemic lupus erythematosus, drug eruption, toxic epidermal necrolysis, erythema multiforme, zinc-responsive dermatosis and generic dog food dermatosis.

65 (a) Cutaneous lymphosarcoma, tumour stage.
(b) None. This disease is non-responsive to chemotherapy or radiation therapy. Corticosteroids will help to decrease the pruritus and inflammation very temporarily. Antibiotics are somewhat helpful to reduce secondary infection. Most patients are euthanised within 3 months of diagnosis of this form of cutaneous cancer.

66 (a) The most common presenting signs of canine allergic inhalant disease are:
1 Foot licking/chewing with interdigital inflammation. 2 Face rubbing. 3 Otitis externa. 4 Axillary pruritus. 5 Recurrent bacterial skin infections.
(b) Antihistamines are helpful in only mildly allergic patients. Corticosteroids may safely be used in most canine allergic patients for up to 4 months per year. If antihistamines are not helpful, and unsafe levels of corticosteroids are needed to control the patient's discomfort, intradermal allergy testing and hyposensitization (immunotherapy) are recommended. The serum tests for inhalant allergies (ELISA, RAST) are considered by most dermatologic allergists to be less reliable than intradermal testing.
(c) Many breeds appear to be predisposed. They are now too numerous to list. It seems to be that when a breed of dog becomes very popular there is indiscriminate breeding, which predisposes the breed to genetic abnormalities.

67 Coccidioidomycosis. This is a systemic fungal infection of dogs and cats in the southwestern United States. Primary skin lesions are rare, although skin lesions may be seen in disseminated cases.

68 (a) Female sex hormone hypersensitivity.
(b) Differential diagnoses include flea bite hypersensitivity, food hypersensitivity, intestinal parasite hypersensitivity, drug hypersensitivity, allergic inhalant disease (atopy) and ovarian imbalance type I.
(c) Definitive diagnosis is made by thorough history-taking, complete physical examination, intradermal skin testing using aqueous sex hormones and response to therapy. Intradermal skin testing is performed with aqueous progesterone (0.025 mg), oestrogen (0.0125 mg) and testosterone (0.05 mg). The skin test sites are observed for immediate (10-minute) and delayed (48 – 72-hour) hypersensitivity reactions.
Note: The aqueous hormones may be difficult to obtain; therefore, the diagnosis may need to be made by a favourable response to ovariohysterectomy.

69 (a) *Dermatophilus congolensis*.
(b) Dermatophillosis. This is a rare disease of the dog and cat and is seen most commonly in moist, warm climates.
(c) Treatment includes the elimination of the primary inciting factors such as moisture, ectoparasites and/or skin trauma. Crusts should be gently removed from the skin and the patient bathed with a mild povidone iodine or chlorhexidine-containing shampoo. Topical lime-sulphur 'dips' are also helpful. Therapy with high levels of tetracycline or penicillin for 7 – 14 days is usually curative.

70 (a) Usually solitary.
(b) Yes. American Cocker spaniels.
(c) The lesions may recur at the site of surgical excision, but they rarely metastasize.
(d) Face and head.

71 (a) Hyperthyroidism. The most common clinical signs of hyperthyroidism in the cat are not dermatologic. They include weight loss, diarrhoea, irritability, increased vocalisation and bizarre behaviour patterns. Some patients will excessively groom themselves and present with self-induced alopecia.
(b) Elevated resting serum thyroid levels, total T4 and free T4, are usually diagnostic.
(c) Treatment options include surgical removal of the abnormal thyroid gland, and oral administration of tapazole (which must be closely monitored).

72 (a) Hypotestosteronism or testosterone-responsive alopecia.
(b) Methyl-testosterone, orally, at a dosage of 0.25 mg per pound of body weight, every other day for 90 days. After the hair has regrown, once-weekly administration of the drug is usually sufficient. (Do not exceed the recommended dose, nor use this drug with cats, as it may cause liver disease and/or irreversible bone marrow suppression.)

73 (a) Feline tail (preen) gland hyperplasia, 'stud tail'.
(b) Therapy includes the use of benzoyl peroxide shampoos (which act as follicular flushing agents, but must be used at a concentration of less than 3%), anti-seborrhoeic shampoos which do not contain tar, and topical Retin-A. Corticosteroids definitely have significant, short-term benefit. The condition is usually a chronic one; however, as most of these patients age, the frequency of recurrences decreases.

74 (a) Parasitic skin disease, namely dirofilaria immitus and/or dipetalonema. (This skin condition is rare in the dog. However, numerous cases of exudative, non-healing, sometimes nodular lesions have been reported in dogs with heartworm disease. No direct cause and effect relationship has ever been documented.)

(b)   A blood sample should be examined for heartworm larvae.

75 (a)   Haemangiosarcoma.
(b)   In the spleen.
(c)   The liver, lungs and right atrial appendage of the heart. The cutaneous lesions in this patient represent metastases from the primary tumour in the spleen.

76 (a)   Urticaria, secondary to a bee sting(s).
(b)   Occasionally, dogs with urticaria may progress to an angio-oedematous reaction involving the nasal passages, pharynx and larynx which could be fatal. Also, some dogs with urticarial lesions progress to anaphylactic shock.
(c)   Pruritus may or may not be present in these reactions.

77 (a)   Hyperplastic dermatosis of the West Highland White terrier (epidermal dysplasia of the West Highland White terrier, 'westie' seborrhoeic disease, and 'westie' armadillo syndrome).
(b)   Sarcoptic mange, demodectic mange, early-onset allergic inhalant disease (atopy) and food hypersensitivity.
(c)   Diagnosis is based upon the breed of the patient, the age of onset of clinical signs (less than one year of age), skin biopsies submitted for histopathologic examination and ruling out the differentials listed in (b) above. Skin biopsies reveal severe acanthosis and mild hyperkeratosis. The epidermis in some patients shows dysplastic changes such as increased mitotic index and uneven nuclear size.
(d)   Treatment is very difficult and very frustrating. The treatment of secondary bacterial and yeast (*Malassezia* spp.) infections is quite important. Corticosteroids relieve some of the pruritus and help to decrease abnormal sebaceous gland secretion, but are usually required at potentially unsafe dosages. Anti-seborrhoeic shampoos are of temporary benefit.
Note: The ketoconazole used to treat the secondary yeast infections in these patients may have some effect in normalising keratinisation. The dosage is 6 – 10 mg per kg of body weight once daily for 15 – 30 days.

78 (a)   Hypothyroidism.
(b)   Ideally, confirmation is by TSH (thyroid stimulating hormone) tests. Other appropriate tests are resting levels of total T4, free T4, total T3 and free T3.
(c)   The 'sad' expression (tragic facies) is caused by myxoedema (mucinous degeneration) with increased dermal mucin deposition.

79 (a)   Malignant melanoma.
(b)   This tumour commonly metastasizes via the lymphatics to the regional (mandibular) lymph nodes. More widespread metastasis to the lungs and other organs is not uncommon in cases of malignant melanoma in the dog.

80 (a)   Common.
(b)   Usually less than 1cm in diameter.
(c)   They may be either solitary or multiple.

81 (a)   Bacterial skin infection, bullous autoimmune skin disease (such as canine pemphigoid), systemic lupus erythematosus and urticaria.
(b)   Eliminate the apparent causative drug (sulpha antibiotic), supportive care and anti-inflammatory doses of corticosteroids.

82 (a)   Traction alopecia caused by repeated use of rubber bands and hair clips to keep the hair out of the patient's eyes.
(b)   None. The alopecia is permanent. (For cosmetic purposes the alopecic area may be

surgically removed under local anaesthesia.)

83 (a) Canine familial dermatomyositis.
(b) Clinical signs, age of patient and breed of dog are important, but the most important diagnostic tool is histopathologic examination of multiple skin biopsies.
(c) Shetland sheepdog and collie.

84 (a) Male sex hormone-responsive alopecia and adult-onset growth hormone deficiency (growth hormone-responsive alopecia).
(b) Pomeranian, Chow Chow, Samoyed, Keeshond and Miniature Poodle.

85 (a) The louse *Felicola subrostrata*.
(b) All cats in contact with this kitten must be treated. The kitten should be washed in a cleansing shampoo, and a topical insecticide applied (lime-sulphur dips, pyrethrim dips) weekly for at least 4 weeks.
(c) The owner should be informed that this is a highly contagious disease for other cats. The louse is species specific, therefore family dogs need not be treated. The louse is incapable of living in the environment for any significant amount of time. Since lice are species specific, this is not a zoonotic disease.

86 (a) Canine haemangiopericytoma. On cytologic examination, the tumour cells are fusiform in their morphology.
(b) By amputation of the limb.
(c) Canine hemangiopericytomas rarely metastasize (less than 0.5% of cases). However, they very frequently recur at the site of surgical excision.

87 (a) Nasal cryptococcosis. *Cryptococcus neoformans* is a saprophyte that can invade the nasal cavities and skin of dogs and cats. It is a common cause of chronic sinusitis, nasal discharge and nasal masses in cats, and can present as multiple cutaneous nodules.
(b) Itraconazole.

88 (a) Ehlers–Danlos syndrome, cutaneous aesthenia, rubber puppy syndrome.
(b) None. Great care must be taken when handling, grooming, and treating these patients.

89 (a) Cutaneous horn.
(b) By wide surgical excision.

90 (a) Pemphigus vulgaris, systemic lupus erythematosus and toxic epidermal necrolysis.
(b) Biopsies for histopathologic examination, biopsies for direct immunofluorescence testing (positive) and ANA—antinuclear antibody testing (positive).
(c) Systemic lupus erythematosus.
(d) Yes.
Comments: Systemic lupus erythematosus is an uncommon-to-rare disease of the dog and cat. In dogs, the German shepherd dog, collie, Shetland sheepdog and Poodle may be predisposed. There is no feline breed predisposition. Since approximately only 20% of patients show cutaneous abnormalities, signs of other organ disease are quite important.

91 Bilateral renal cystadenocarcinoma, uterine leiomyoma.
Note: The editor has seen many cases of German shepherd dog nodular dermatofibrosis unassociated with any other neoplastic disease.

92 (a) Furuncle, furunculosis.
(b) Bacterial (most commonly *Staphylococcus intermedius*), fungal (dermatophytosis) and parasitic (demodicosis). Furunculosis is most commonly caused by bacteria.

(c) Localised furunculosis may involve the chin, muzzle, pressure point callouses, bridge of the nose and the interdigital spaces. Dogs (especially German shepherd dogs) may also develop a generalised furunculosis.

93 (a) Feline eosinophilic plaque, secondary to an underlying pruritic skin disease (allergy).
(b) The clinical appearance of these lesions is quite helpful. However, a biopsy submitted for histopathologic examination is the only way to confirm this diagnosis.
(c) Recurrent eosinophilic plaques in the feline that are corticosteroid-responsive are almost always due to one or more of the following:
1 Flea bite allergy. 2 Food hypersensitivity. 3 Allergic inhalant disease (atopy).

94 (a) 1 Demodicosis. 2 Dermatophytosis. 3 Bacterial pyoderma. 4 Pemphigus foliaceus.
5 Zinc dermatopathy. 6 Generic dog food dermatosis.
(b) What is this dog being fed?
(c) 1 Skin scrapings for demodectic mites would be negative. 2 A fungal culture would be negative. 3 Skin biopsies submitted for histopathologic examination reveal a moderate parakeratosis, occasional dyskeratosis, occasional necrolytic areas of the superficial epidermis, with a slightly acanthotic epidermis.
(d) The cutaneous abnormalities, negative skin scrapings and fungal culture, biopsy results and the fact that the pup is being fed a sub-standard, unbalanced diet are diagnostic for generic dog food dermatosis.

95 (a) Eosinophilic ulcer, feline rodent ulcer.
(b) A carefully taken skin biopsy for histopathologic examination is the diagnostic test of choice.
(c) The initial treatment is glucocorticoids. Cats typically respond most favourably to subcutaneous or intramuscular methyl prednisolone acetate at a dosage of 5 mg per kg of body weight. This may be repeated every 2 – 3 weeks for a total of three treatments, then every 3 months. Cats are much less responsive to the administration of oral cortisone. (The injectable methyl prednisolone acetate may cause temporary or permanent diabetes mellitus in some cats.)
(d) Allergic inhalant disease (atopy), food hypersensitivity, flea bite allergy. Much less commonly these patients will be FIV or FeLV positive.

96 (a) Erythema multiforme.
(b) Bacterial folliculitis, dermatophytosis, demodicosis, systemic lupus erythematosus, pemphigus vulgaris, bullous pemphigoid, mycoses fungoides and other vesicular and pustular skin diseases.
(c) This patient's erythema multiforme is probably due to an adverse reaction to the penicillin. Erythema multiforme has also been reported to be caused by bacterial and viral infections, so it is possible that the patient's respiratory infection was the inciting cause.

97 (a) German shepherd dog furunculosis, folliculitis and cellulitis; deep pyoderma of the German shepherd dog.
(b) *Staphylococcus intermedius* is the most common organism, although haemolytic streptococci, *Escherichia coli* and coagulase-negative staphylococci have also been cultured from these patients.
(c) Often the initial clinical sign reported by the owners is pruritus.
(d) The prognosis for 'cure' is not good. The skin disease often relapses after long-term systemic antibiotic therapy (6 – 12 weeks) is discontinued. In recurrent cases, it is essential to check carefully for underlying factors that may cause pruritus and/or the decreased ability of the skin to fight off bacterial infection. These include flea bite hypersensitivity, intestinal parasitism and hypothyroidism. If recurrences still occur, staphylococcal bacterin therapy, immune

and hypothyroidism. If recurrences still occur, staphylococcal bacterin therapy, immune modulation, or long-term, lower dose antibiotics (once daily, or several times weekly) may be used.

98 (a) Generalised demodicosis, demodectic mange.
(b) Because of the secondary bacterial skin infection, a 4 – 6 week course of systemic antibiotics is indicated. Antihistamines may be helpful in decreasing the pruritus. (Corticosteroids are contra-indicated in patients with demodicosis.) The most important part of the therapy is weekly amitrax dips until the owners feel that the patient appears to have normal skin. Once this point is reached, the patient should again be skin scraped in at least 10 different areas. If any mites (dead, alive or eggs) are present, the owners are sent home with 6 more dips to be applied at weekly intervals. The patient is again presented for repeat, multiple skin scrapings. The dippings are not stopped until all mites are eliminated. (The editor feels that most cases of 'recurrent' demodicosis in young dogs are not really recurrences, but that the mites were never really eliminated in the first place. Following this treatment protocol, the editor reports greater than a 95% cure rate.)
(c) The owners should first be informed that the disease is hereditary and that affected dogs (males and females) should not be used in any breeding programme. They should be neutered as soon as the demodicosis is somewhat under control. The owners should also be informed that this is a difficult, expensive and time-consuming treatment protocol. The owners must be willing to follow the treatment instructions exactly, or it is not worth the effort even to initiate therapy.

99 (a) Cutaneous melanoma. Miniature Schnauzers are predisposed to the development of cutaneous melanomas. Most of these arise on the back, neck and thorax.
(b) Cutaneous melanomas are considered to be benign tumours in the dog, especially when they arise from haired skin. However, all melanomas should be submitted for histopathologic examination to differentiate the benign tumours from the malignant tumours. Benign versus malignant is based primarily on the microscopic mitotic activity.
Note: Although the miniature Schnauzer is also predisposed to the development of cutaneous malignant melanomas, only one tumour in eight is malignant, and these arise primarily on the forelimbs.

100 (a) Bullous (canine) pemphigoid, pemphigus vulgaris, systemic lupus erythematosus, toxic epidermal necrolysis, hidradenitis suppurativa and ulcerative dermatosis of the collie and Shetland sheepdog.
(b) Skin biopsies for histopathologic examination.
(c) Ulcerative dermatosis of the collie and Shetland sheepdog.

101 (a) Very rare. It is estimated that less than 100 Sphinx cats reside in the United States.
(b) Yes. This breed has very excessive sebum and cerumin production, usually requiring daily bathing and ear cleaning.

102 (a) Nasal pyoderma is most commonly seen in the German shepherd dog, collie, Pointer and 'hunting-type' (dolichocephalic) breeds. The underlying aetiology is not known.
(b) Differential diagnoses include: immune-mediated (autoimmune) diseases such as discoid lupus erythematosus, systemic lupus erythematosus, pemphigus foliaceus, demodicosis, dermatophytosis, drug eruptions, dermatomyositis, trauma and solar dermatitis.
(c) Clinical management includes consideration of the underlying causes and systemic antibiotic therapy. A short course of corticosteroids is quite important in decreasing the pain and inflammation, as well as decreasing the chances of permanent scarring of the nose. Systemic antibiotics are usually required for 3 – 6 weeks. This disorder, unlike other bacterial skin

infections, does not usually recur. However, permanent scarring of the bridge of the nose, with permanent alopecia, is a common sequela.

103 (a) Dalmatian bronzing syndrome and staphylococcal folliculitis. It was previously believed that the bronzing seen in many Dalmatians with this condition was related to their unusual protein metabolism and the resultant elevated uric acid levels. This belief has not been proven, and it is now thought that this bronze discolouration is the result of the bacterial folliculitis.
(b) Therapy consists of an appropriate skin antibiotic for 3 – 6 weeks. If the patient was being fed a high protein diet, the diet should be changed to one containing normal protein levels. (Some patients respond very favourably to commercially prepared 'vegetarian' diets.)

104 (a) Linear granuloma. This is a common cutaneous disease of cats. It may present as this 'classic' granuloma (pictured), or as nodules on the chin, lips and ears. The cause is unknown, but is suspected to be of allergic aetiology.
(b) The treatment of choice is parenteral glucocorticoids such as methyl prednisolone acetate at a dosage of 5 mg/kg of body weight, administered intramuscularly or subcutaneously. This may need to be repeated in 2 – 6 weeks. The cat is much less responsive to oral glucocorticoids than is the dog.
(c) The prognosis for this patient is excellent. Many linear granulomas in cats less than one year of age will spontaneously regress over several months.

105 (a) Cutaneous lymphangioma.
(b) Wide surgical excision is the treatment of choice.
(c) This prognosis is guarded. This tumour commonly recurs at the site of surgical excision due to its infiltrative nature as well as the difficulty in macroscopically identifying surgical borders.

106 (a) Canine eosinophilic granuloma.
(b) Any age, breed, or sex of dog may develop this disease. However, 80% of cases occur in dogs less than 3 years old; 76% occur in Siberian huskies; and 72% occur in males.
(c) Eosinophilic granulomas in the dog occur most commonly in the oral cavity and present as ulcerated palatine plaques and vegetative lingual masses. Less commonly, they occur as multiple, cutaneous papules, nodules and/or plaques involving the ventral abdomen, prepuce and flanks. The cutaneous lesions are usually non-pruritic and non-painful. The patients are otherwise healthy. The aetiology of these lesions is not known; however, a hypersensitivity reaction or vasculopathy is a reported pathogenic mechanism.

107 (a) Nasal hyperkeratosis.
(b) The footpads.
(c) No treatment is really necessary unless the condition causes discomfort to the dog. This occasionally happens in severe cases in which the nose fissures and bleeds. Sometimes it is a disease of significant cosmetic concern to the patient's owner. If the dog is uncomfortable, or if the owner wishes, treatment may be initiated. Topicals of possible benefit include ointments containing salicylic acid, lactic acid and/or corticosteroids. However, most normal dogs will not allow these products to remain on their noses for any useful amount of time. The retinoid etretinate may be prescribed systemically, although its benefit is questionable and potential side effects must be monitored. (The editor has found that the use of a sand-paper 'dremmel' rotary tool to remove the abnormal nose tissue is of the most benefit. This may need to be repeated every 6 – 12 months. Also, a small percentage of these patients are hypothyroid, and correction of this condition helps the nose disease.)
(d) The disease is most commonly seen in American Cocker spaniels, Springer spaniels and brachycephalic breeds of dogs.

108 (a) *Notoedres cati*. It is often called 'feline scabies'. On microscopic examination, the mite is quite similar to both the canine and the human scabies mite. This mite is highly contagious for other felines and usually causes intense pruritus. The most common site of intense pruritus is the head. The mite may cause a transient pruritic dermatitis on canine and human skin. However, the mite is species specific and is incapable of completing its life cycle on dogs, humans and other species.

(b) Because this infestation is highly contagious, the affected cat should be isolated from other cats until the mites are eliminated. All cats who have been in contact with the infested cat should be treated with an appropriate miticide, such as lime sulphur dips weekly for 8 weeks, or subcutaneous ivermectin every 2 weeks for four treatments. (Other species need not be treated.) Finally, it is quite helpful to try to identify the original source of the infestation. If this is not done, re-infestation is likely to occur. (Apparently, the premises need not be treated because the mite is incapable of living off the host.)

109 (a) Inflammatory polyp.

(b) The middle ear.

(c) The lesions may also be found in the pharyngeal area. In these cases, the mass grows from the middle ear down the eustachian tube.

110 (a) Human flea bite dermatitis. The feet are a very common location of flea bites in humans.

(b) Sarcoptic mange (*Sarcoptes scabiei* var. *canis*)—the canine scabies mite is capable of causing an intensely pruritic papular dermatitis in humans. *Cheyletiella* mite—this mite may cause very pruritic papules in humans exposed to animals infested with *Cheyletiella* or in humans in infested environments. The *Cheyletiella* mite may live in the environment for several days.

111 (a) Multiple skin biopsies for histopathologic examination are usually diagnostic.

(b) Nodular dermatofibrosis (multiple dermal fibromas).

(c) Renal epithelial neoplasia (bilateral renal cystadenoma).

(d) Yes, highly predisposed.

(e) There is no known effective treatment.

112 (a) Muzzle folliculitis/furunculosis, canine chin acne.

(b) Chin acne is most commonly seen in young dogs (less than one year of age), and in short-coated breeds of dogs (usually the larger ones). Common breeds of dogs affected with this condition include the Boxer, Dobermann pinscher, bulldog, Mastiff, Bull mastiff, Great Dane, Weimaraner, and German short-haired pointer. The male dog definitely appears to be predisposed.

(c) Therapy may be limited to benign observation, as many of these cases are innocuous and self-limiting and disappear at the time of, or just after, puberty. It is quite important to rule out demodicosis and dermatophytosis as underlying inciting causes. Benzoyl peroxide, as a gel or shampoo, may be used for its anti-bacterial and follicular-flushing properties. Systemic antibiotics are indicated in severe cases that are not improving with topical therapy. Systemic corticosteroids (for short periods of time) may be necessary to prevent permanent cosmetic defects, such as scarring and alopecia.

113 (a) Feline plasma cell pododermatitis.

(b) The diagnosis is made based upon physical examination, aspiration cytology, culture and biopsies submitted for histopathologic examination.

(c) The therapy of choice is not known, as some cases will regress spontaneously. Also, many cats are asymptomatic and will not require therapy. When treatment is necessary, two courses of therapy have been shown to be effective. The first is relatively high dosages of systemic glucocorticoids (methyl-prednisolone acetate subcutaneously at a dosage of 4 – 5 mg per kg of body weight every 2 – 3 weeks for three treatments. The second is intramuscular gold salt injections (crysotherapy) weekly for 6 – 12 weeks, then monthly if necessary.

114 (a) Bacterial skin infection, subcorneal pustular dermatosis, pemphigus foliaceus and pemphigus vegetans.
(b) Pustule cytology, biopsies for histopathologic examination and skin scrapings. (The histopath biopsies reveal intraepidermal microabscesses which contain mainly eosinophils and acantholytic keratinocytes.)
(c) Pemphigus vegetans.
(d) Extremely rare.
(e) No.

115 (a) (3). No skin disease. This is a normal cat.
(b) Devon Rex.

116 (a) Dermatophyte infection ('ringworm'). The most common organisms that a small animal veterinary technician would be exposed to are *Microsporum canis* and *Trichophyton mentagrophytes*. (This lesion was caused by *Trichophyton mentagrophytes*.)
(b) Exposure to a dog or cat having either a clinical or sub-clinical infection. Statistically, cats are the more common source of human dermatophyte infections.

117 (a) *Cheyletiella* spp.
(b) No. The cause of pruritus in the owner's dogs is most likely due to *Cheyletiella* infestation also.
(c) It would be quite helpful to have the hair coats of all of the pets clipped short. The *Cheyletiella* mite attaches its eggs to the hair, and clipping will remove one source of contagion. All pets in the home should be treated with a topical miticidal dip, such as lime sulphur, amitraz, pyrethrin or malathion. The dippings should be done weekly for 8 weeks. In addition, the home environment should be sprayed with a product formulated to kill fleas. The *Cheyletiella* mite is capable of living in the environment for several weeks.
(d) This mite frequently bites human contacts, causing an intensely pruritic papular dermatitis. It is therefore a zoonotic disease.

118 (a) Feline acne.
(b) Usually the diagnosis is made based upon clinical evaluation. However, a skin biopsy taken for histopathologic examination would show hair follicular distension with prominent sebaceous glands. (The prominent sebaceous glands are normal for the chin area.) Follicular rupture with associated furunculosis may be present.

119 (a) Feline self-induced alopecia.
(b) 1 Flea bite hypersensitivity. 2 Allergic inhalant disease (atopy). 3 Food hypersensitivity. 4 Neurodermatitis (feline psychogenic alopecia).
(c) The most valuable diagnostic test is already listed in the description of the patient's condition. This is the microscopic examination of the stubbly hairs in the affected area to prove that the alopecia is self-induced. Most owners do not observe excessive grooming or licking of the area by their pet. (Cats are often 'closet' lickers!) Once the alopecia is determined to be self-induced (and 99% of cases are), the diagnostic tests of significance are response to flea control (even in the absence of flea evidence), response to a low-allergen diet, and, lastly, intradermal allergy testing for allergic inhalant disease.

120 (a) Proliferative otitis externa. The three most common breeds of dog that appear to be predisposed are the American Cocker spaniel, the English Springer spaniel and the Chinese Shar pei.

(b)   A complete history is essential. This disease is almost always associated with an underlying disease such as allergic inhalant disease (atopy), food hypersensitivity, hypothyroidism, and/or primary keratinisation or sebaceous gland defects. It is very helpful to radiograph the tympanic bullae and external ear canals. Chronic otitis externa is often accompanied by a middle ear infection. Radiographic evaluation of the ear canals is useful in determining whether or not medical management is possible. If the external ear canals are calcified, the patient is not a candidate for medical therapy and surgery should be considered.

(c)   If the ear canals do not show radiographic evidence of calcification, the patient may respond to large doses of oral prednisolone (2 – 5 mg/kg of body weight daily for 7 – 10 days, then every other day for several weeks). This aggressive systemic glucocorticoid therapy will reduce the otic sebaceous proliferation. Concurrent systemic antibiotics are often helpful. Once the extreme swelling of the external ear canal has decreased, topical therapy can be initiated. Once the patient is responding, it is essential to look for and treat the underlying aetiology. If the ear canals are calcified, total ear ablation may be the only effective and humane treatment for these patients.

121   Perianal fistulas, anal sac abscesses and perianal tumours.

122   (a)   Pattern baldness of the short-haired Dachshund, pattern alopecia.

(b)   This condition is seen almost exclusively in Dachshunds. In most cases, diagnosis is based upon clinical evaluation. Confirmation may be obtained by skin biopsies taken for histopathologic examination. Biopsies are not recommended to be taken from ear pinnae, as permanent scarring is a common sequela. However, histopathology does reveal small hair bulbs, but not a predominance of telogen follicles, as would be seen in an endocrinopathy.

(c)   There really is no treatment and the hair loss is usually permanent. However, if the patient is also hypothyroid, correction of this condition may result in some hair regrowth. (The editor has treated many cases with topical minoxidil and some hair re-growth has occurred in about 40% of the patients.)

123   (a)   Idiopathic lichenoid dermatosis, seborrhoeic plaques, and linear verrucous epidermal nevus.

(b)   Multiple skin biopsies taken for histopathologic examination.

(c)   Idiopathic lichenoid dermatosis.

(d)   No form of therapy has been shown to be beneficial in most cases. Systemic corticosteroids decrease inflammation but do not cause regression of the lesions. Retinoid therapy may be beneficial but this has not been used in a significant number of cases. The prognosis is good, because many cases undergo spontaneous remission after a course of 6 – 24 months.

124   (a)   Idiopathic mucinosis of the Chinese Shar pei.

(b)   The fluid is mucin.

(c)   Therapy often is not needed. These patients tend to 'deflate' as they mature (often to the disappointment of their owners). In severe cases, especially if the patient is pruritic, either from this 'primary condition' or from allergic dermatitis, glucocorticoid therapy is usually beneficial. The major benefit is to decrease the pruritus, which can be quite damaging and easily causes ulceration to this vesicular epidermis.

125   (a)   Nasal solar dermatitis. This is an actinic reaction which occurs on poorly pigmented nasal skin of dogs and cats who are frequently exposed to direct sunlight for prolonged periods of time.

(b)   If the lesions are not monitored, and the patient's exposure to sunlight is not limited, the

condition often progresses to deep ulcerations which bleed easily. In advanced cases, squamous cell carcinoma may develop.
(c) Discoid lupus erythematosus, systemic lupus erythematosus, pemphigus erythematosus, pemphigus foliaceus and demodicosis.

126 (a) Pododermatitis, interdigital pyoderma, interdigital 'cysts'.
(b) Demodicosis, dermatophytosis, irritating chemicals, allergic inhalant disease (atopy), obesity, hypothyroidism, intestinal parasites, external parasites (ticks), clipper burns from grooming procedures, housing on wire or on rough stones, immune deficiency disorders and 'idiopathic'.

127 (a) Anal sac gland carcinoma. This tumour arises from the modified apocrine glands of the anal sacs.
(b) The polyuria, polydipsia and weakness are due to a pseudohypoparathyroidism that is commonly found in association with these tumours. This is due to the release of a parathyroid-like hormone by the tumour cells. Difficulty in defecation is often due to tumour metastasis to the sacral lymph node, which impinges upon the underlying rectum.

128 (a) Pelodera dermatitis due to the 'straw itch mite', *Pelodera strongyloides*. The non-seasonal nature of this disease (occurring in an area where there is significant seasonal variation in temperature), and the size of the nematode are inconsistent with hookworm dermatitis. Furthermore, this nematode is a common inhabitant of straw, and dogs bedded on straw that becomes moist are predisposed to this disease.
(b) The most important part of the treatment is to remove the 'contaminated' straw from the dog's environment. The straw should be burned (if possible) and the dog's area thoroughly cleaned and then sprayed with an insecticide that is approved and effective as a premise spray for fleas. Cedar shavings (which may cause contact dermatitis in some dogs), shredded newspaper, or cloth should be used as an alternate bedding. The dog should be bathed, then an insecticidal dip applied weekly for 8 weeks. Subcutaneous ivermectin is also effective but dosages and breed precautions must be carefully observed. Oral and short-acting injectable glucocorticoids are quite effective in decreasing the patient's discomfort. However, in general the disease is self-eliminating if the infected bedding is removed.

129 Pruritus in dogs with hyperadrenocorticism (Cushing's disease) is not common. It is usually associated with the presence of secondary bacterial skin infection, seborrhoeic abnormalities, demodicosis and/or calcinosis cutis.

130 (a) Sertoli-cell tumour, less commonly seminoma or interstitial cell tumour.
(b) Castration is definitely the treatment of choice.
(c) Prior to surgery, thoracic radiographs should be taken and evaluated for metastasis. A complete blood and platelet count should be performed to check for anaemia and thrombocytopenia, which have occasionally been associated with Sertoli-cell tumours. Both of these abnormalities could easily lead to surgical complications.

131 (a) Sebaceous adenitis.
(b) Skin biopsies submitted in 10% buffered formalin for histopathologic examination.
(c) Various treatments have been reported to improve this (hereditary?) skin disease, but there is no cure. A topical solution of 50% propylene glycol sprayed on the abnormal coat every 1 – 2 days is helpful, but quite messy. Glucocorticoids decrease the inflammation, decrease the pruritus (if it exists) and help to decrease the abnormal sebaceous gland function. Synthetic retinoids have been helpful in some patients, but are expensive and must be closely monitored for side effects.

Note: Until more is learned about this disease, affected canines should not be used in breeding programmes.

132 (a) Autoimmune skin disease, specifically pemphigus foliaceus.
(b) Biopsies for histopathologic examination (which are often diagnostic), biopsies for direct immunofluorescence (usually positive), antinuclear antibody testing (negative) and skin scrapings (negative for demodectic mites).
Comments: Pemphigus foliaceus is the most common autoimmune skin disease seen in the dog and cat.

133 (a) Hormonal imbalances (which include hypothyroidism, male sex hormone-responsive alopecia and hyperadrenocorticism) and canine follicular dysplasia (idiopathic flank alopecia).
(b) Canine follicular dysplasia of the miniature Schnauzer.
(c) English bulldogs, Boxers, Airedale terriers and French bulldogs.

134 (a) Very rare.
(b) Less than 18 months of age.
(c) The miniature and standard short-haired Dachshund exclusively.
Note: Axillary hyperpigmentation, lichenification and seborrhoeic dermatitis are common clinical signs in many breeds of dogs. However, these skin changes are always secondary to an underlying skin disease. (See secondary acanthosis nigricans.)

135 (a) Cutaneous lymphosarcoma.
(b) 'Pautrier microabscess' is an intra-epidermal aggregation of neoplastic lymphoid cells found in the epidermotrophic form of cutaneous lymphosarcoma. They are not present in the tumours that are non-epidermotrophic.

136 (a) Hookworm dermatitis. Skin scrapings of the feet are usually negative in affected dogs. However, the history of a common exercise pen, in which the faeces are not removed daily, classic clinical signs, and a faecal flotation positive for hookworm ova are strongly supportive of this diagnosis. Hookworm larvae are capable of penetrating human skin in contact with the contaminated grassy areas.
(b) All dogs should be treated with an appropriate anthelmintic. The premises must be thoroughly cleansed and a daily faecal-pick-up programme instituted. Borax may be applied to contaminated surfaces to kill hookworm larvae, but it will also kill the vegetation. Other larvacides are available.

137 (a) Feline cutaneous mast cell tumour.
(b) Cutaneous haemangioma and cutaneous lymphangioma.
(c) Neoplastic mast cells, either singly or aggregated in small groups.
(d) An extensive amount of mucinous matrix may be associated with some mast cell tumours, giving them a soft feel.

138 (a) Vitamin A-'responsive' dermatosis.
(b) Vitamin A supplementation at a dosage of 10,000 I.U. 1 – 2 times daily may show improvement in 8 – 12 weeks. If so, then the dose is significantly reduced. Unfortunately, many of these Cockers whose skin biopsies show a vitamin A-responsive dermatopathy do not respond to this regime of supplementation. Some patients respond to the much more expensive, synthetic vitamin A derivatives such as etretinate and isotretinoin; some Cockers do not respond to any forms of vitamin A, and palliative therapy is necessary. This includes keratinolytic shampoos, systemic antibiotics (when indicated), and oral glucocorticoid to decrease itch and inflammation.

139 (a) Vitiligo. Pigment loss in skin is called leucoderma; in hair it is called leucotrichia.
(b) Rottweilers, Dobermann pinschers, Belgian Tervurens and German shepherd dogs.

140 (a) Interdigital sterile pyogranulomas are most common in smooth, short-coated breeds of dog such as English bulldogs, short-haired Dachshunds, Great Danes, Boxers, Mastiffs and English mastiffs.
(b) Systemic, short-acting, oral corticosteroids (prednisone, prednisolone) at a dosage of 2.2 mg per kg of body weight once daily until the lesion(s) is dramatically improved are the most effective therapy. Then the dosage is reduced to alternate day therapy, and should be reduced or stopped as indicated by the patient's response.
Note: Hypothyroidism should be ruled out.

141 (a) Squamous cell carcinoma.
(b) Excessive exposure to short-wave ultraviolet light (UVB). Chronic sun exposure induces epithelial changes due to clonal mutation and damage to the keratinocytes.

142 (a) The patient's history and the location of the lesions are highly suggestive of frostbite.
(b) The lesions should be gently cleansed and handled with care. It is often difficult to assess the extent of damage visually. Necrotic tissue should be debrided and the lesions treated similarly to a burn. In severe cases the ear pinnal tips require surgical removal.

143 (a) Feline tail gland hyperplasia or 'stud tail'.
(b) This diagnosis is usually a clinical one, made after examination of the patient, careful history taking, negative skin scrapings, fungal culture and no evidence of parasites. However, a definitive diagnosis may be made via skin biopsies submitted for histopathologic examination in 10% buffered formalin. (We must always ask: if the skin lesion created by the diagnostic test and the associated trauma is worse than the disease we are attempting to diagnose, is the diagnostic test really in the best interest of the patient?) When skin biopsies are performed, they reveal sebaceous gland hyperplasia, as well as follicular distension with rupture of the hair follicle and occasionally an associated bacterial furunculosis.
(c) Treatment usually involves cleansing the tail, gently, with a 3% benzoyl peroxide shampoo and the use of systemic glucocorticoids (an injection of methyl prednisolone acetate at a dosage of 4 – 5 mg/kg). Occasionally, systemic antibiotics will be necessary. If the patient is an intact male cat, neutering may be beneficial, but it must be remembered that most cases do not involve intact male cats!

144 (a) Linear prepucial dermatosis.
(b) This skin change is associated with hyperoestrogenism in male dogs. The most common causes are Sertoli-cell tumour and interstitial cell tumour. However, it has been seen with exogenous oestrogen administration.

145 (a) Demodectic mange, pemphigus erythematosus and foliaceus, systemic lupus erythematosus, dermatophyte infection.
(b) Skin scrapings for demodectic mites, fungal culture, punch biopsies for histopathologic examination (in 10% buffered formalin) and punch biopsies for direct immunofluorescence testing (in Michel's media).
(c) Pemphigus foliaceus.
(d) No.
(e) Yes. Approximately 60% of patients live relatively normal lives with therapy.
(f) Corticosteroids, azathioprine and injectable gold salts.

146 (a) Acral lick dermatitis, acral pruritic nodules.
(b) Allergic inhalant disease or atopy.

147 (a)   Cutaneous haemangioma and cutaneous melanoma.
(b)   Cytologic examination of an aspirate or an impression smear of the mass is quite helpful.
(c)   Both are best treated by wide surgical excision.
(d)   Both tumours have a good prognosis. However, histologic examination is essential to differentiate these tumours from cutaneous haemangiosarcomas and cutaneous malignant melanomas.

148 (a)   Secondary acanthosis nigricans.
(b)   Food hypersensitivity, hormonal hypersensitivity, flea bite allergy, contact dermatitis, hypothyroidism, various sex hormone 'imbalances', primary seborrhoeic disorders such as those seen in the Cocker spaniel, and constant friction in the axillary areas caused by obesity or conformational abnormalities.

149 (a)   Cutaneous tag.
(b)   The lesion is also referred to as a skin tag, acrochordon or fibroepithelial polyp.
(c)   This lesion is benign and is thought to arise due to mild, continuous irritation of the skin. Therefore, it is possible to find similar lesions at other sites of irritation. The major significance of these lesions is their cosmetic appearance and the fact that they are easily traumatised by routine grooming such as combing, brushing and clipping.

150 (a)   Systemic lupus erythematosus, pemphigus vulgaris, toxic epidermal necrolysis.
(b)   Complete blood count, chemistry profile, antinuclear antibody testing, biopsies for histopathologic and immunofluorescence testing.
(c)   Pemphigus vulgaris.
Comments: Pemphigus vulgaris is a very uncommon autoimmune skin disease of the dog and cat. There is no reported age, breed or sex predilection.

151 (a)   No. The Dobermann pinscher, Spitz, Chow Chow, German shepherd dog and Kuvasz have been diagnosed with canine familial dermatomyositis.
(b)   The aetiopathogenesis is not known. Some believe that the disease is a combination of genetic predisposition as well as viral stimulation. Autoimmune components may also be involved.
(c)   Some cases have spontaneous regression. However, some patients suffer from permanent scarring and/or advanced muscle disease. Anti-inflammatory medications, including corticosteroids may be of some benefit. Others feel that immuno-stimulants (since this disease may be viral-based) are beneficial.

152 (a)   No.
(b)   This condition is called preauricular alopecia and is a normal thinning of the hair coat (to varying degrees) in the preauricular areas. It is present to some degree in most cats.

153 (a)   Black hair follicular dysplasia.
(b)   Clinical signs and biopsies for histopathologic examination.
(c)   None. The hair loss in the black areas is progressive and permanent.

154 (a)   Calcinosis cutis caused by exogenous use of systemic glucocorticoids. The amount and duration of glucocorticoids needed to cause calcinosis cutis varies greatly from patient to patient. Some dogs receive 'allergic dosages' of cortisone for years and do not develop calcinosis cutis. Other cases have shown that calcinosis cutis may develop in dogs who have received relatively low dosages of cortisone for several months.
(b)   Confirmation of calcinosis cutis may be made by skin biopsies submitted for histopathologic examination. However, in many cases, the 'bony' feel to the epidermis is diagnostic in itself.

(c) The glucocorticoids must be tapered, then discontinued. Severe cases of calcinosis cutis may take up to 6 months to resolve, either by reabsorption or by transepidermal elimination. Some dogs require surgical excision of the large calcium deposits. (Obviously, it is now necessary to determine which type of allergy is causing this patient's pruritus and attempt to treat this, rather than to treat the itch with cortisone.)

155 (a) Miliary dermatitis, self-induced hair loss and lesions of the eosinophilic granuloma complex.
(b) The most important treatment is elimination of the fleas, both on the cat and in the environment. Subcutaneous methyl-prednisolone acetate (4 – 5 mg/kg of body weight) is quite helpful in reducing pruritus. Oral corticosteroids are less effective in the cat than in the dog. Occasionally, antibiotics are indicated.

156 (a) Discoid lupus erythematosus, Vogt–Koyanagi–Harada-like syndrome, systemic lupus erythematosus and 'Dudley nose'.
(b) Biopsies for histopathologic examination.
(c) 'Dudley nose', nasal leucoderma, collie nose.

157 (a) Angio-oedema.
(b) Anaphylactic shock.
(c) Fortunately this emergency, potentially fatal situation is a very rare sequela to intradermally injected skin test antigens.
(d) A similar anaphylactic response to hyposensitization (immunotherapy).

158 (a) Pemphigus vulgaris, systemic lupus erythematosus, bullous (canine) pemphigoid, toxic epidermal necrolysis, erythema multiforme and ulcerative dermatosis of the collie and Shetland sheepdog.
(b) Ulcerative dermatosis of the collie and Shetland sheepdog.
Comment: This is a newly recognised cutaneous syndrome about which very little is known. The disease is seen in adult collies and Shetland sheepdogs, and usually involves the axillary and inguinal areas and occasionally the oral mucosa. Since myositis has been diagnosed in some patients, this disease may be another manifestation of canine familial dermatomyositis. Biopsies for histopathologic examination, antinuclear antibody testing (negative) and biopsies for direct immunofluorescence testing (negative) are usually able to differentiate this disease from the other differential diagnoses.

159 Flea bite hypersensitivity. Feline allergic inhalant disease (atopy). Food hypersensitivity. *Cheyletiella* infestation. Dermatophytosis. Bacterial folliculitis.

160 The most likely cause is *Cheyletiella* bites. Usually, infested cats are quite pruritic; however, some cats merely exhibit an excessive scale production which is called 'walking dandruff'. The mites are quite easily found on skin scrapings taken from the involved feline. Humans exposed to infested pets often have intensely pruritic papular dermatitis. Since the *Cheyletiella* mites are capable of living in the home environment for several days, treatment of the cat with a parasiticidal dip as well as using a home 'insecticide' are necessary.

161 (a) The differentials include a flare-up of allergic inhalant disease, demodicosis, dermatophyte infection and bacterial skin infection. A skin scraping of the foot or face readily reveals numerous demodectic mites.
(b) This patient will be quite difficult to control because the corticosteroids which are needed to control her allergic inhalant disease (atopy) are exacerbating (or causing) her demodicosis. Most likely she will require lifelong amitraz dips and occasional antibiotics to control her demodicosis. The cortisone will have to be continued because the severity of this patient's

139

allergies causes her to be miserable without it.

162 (a) Feline pemphigus foliaceus.
(b) Rafts of acantholytic cells are seen along with neutrophils. Bacteria are not observed.
(c) The cytologic findings as well as the physical examination are highly suggestive of pemphigus foliaceus. A definitive diagnosis may be made via multiple skin biopsies submitted in 10% buffered formalin for histopathologic examination. Direct immunofluorescence of skin biopsies in Michel's media may be helpful. However, false negatives and false positives are common. (The footpads and noses of many normal dogs and cats show positive fluorescence.)

163 (a) Cutaneous lymphosarcoma.
(b) Skin biopsies taken of numerous lesions and/or nodules.
(c) Regional lymph nodes, spleen and the liver are the most common sites of metastasis.

164 (a) This organism is ubiquitous in the environment and infections are most likely acquired from water or soil.
(b) This organism can invade the gastrointestinal tract, central nervous system and eyes.
(c) This disease is considered to be zoonotic; however, dog-to-human transmission has not been reported. Owners and pets most likely share a common source of exposure.

165 (a) Toxic epidermal necrolysis, pemphigus vulgaris, canine pemphigoid, systemic lupus erythematosus and ulcerative dermatosis of the collie and Shetland sheepdog.
(b) Bullous (canine) pemphigoid.
(c) No.
(d) No.

166 (a) Acral lick dermatitis or acral pruritic nodule.
(b) Osteosarcoma.
(c) Allergic inhalant disease, flea bite allergy, foreign body, hypothyroidism, neuritis, bone or joint pain and boredom.

167 1 Trichoepithelioma (proven on histopathologic examination). 2 Basal cell tumour.
3 Cutaneous melanoma. 4 Squamous cell carcinoma *in situ* (Bowen's disease).

168 (a) Sarcoptic mange, canine scabies.
(b) Multiple skin scrapings (especially of the crusted ear pinnal margins) may reveal the diagnostic mite. However, approximately 40% of canine scabies patients have negative skin scrapings, and therefore history taking and careful physical examination are essential.
(c) Some of the 'conventional' treatments are ineffective in treating current scabies epidemics. The editor has found that subcutaneous Ivermectin (Bovine Ivomec®), given at a dosage of 0.1 cc per 4.5 kg body weight for six treatments every 14 days, is highly effective. This drug cannot be used in collies, Shetland sheepdogs or patients with heartworm disease. In these patients, the treatment of choice is weekly amitraz dips for 6 weeks.
(d) The disease is contracted in several ways. These include:
1 Being boarded at a kennel near a dog who has sarcoptic mange. 2 Being groomed at a grooming parlour that recently groomed a sarcoptic mange patient. 3 Close contact with any dog who has sarcoptic mange. 4 Exposure to areas where infested red foxes have been. These animals often contract a form of crusted sarcoptic mange in which scratched-off scabs containing hundreds of mites may be infective for several days.
(e) Yes. Canine sarcoptic mange can cause an intensely pruritic papular dermatitis in human contacts. The mites are capable of burrowing in human skin, laying eggs, depositing faeces, and having eggs hatch. However, it appears that the life cycle of canine scabies cannot be completed on/in human skin.

169 (a) Feline mast cell tumour.
(b) Wide surgical excision is the treatment of choice for feline mast cell tumours. They are usually benign. There is no evidence that the use of systemic glucocorticoids is helpful in treating or preventing these feline tumours, as is the case in many canine patients.

170 (a) Squamous cell carcinoma.
(b) Malignant melanoma.
(c) Unfortunately, the prognosis is quite difficult to determine. Most of these tumours are solitary, some multiple, and in some studies a significant percentage of metastasis has been reported.

171 (a) Bacterial folliculitis.
(b) The most common aetiologic agent in the cat is coagulase-positive *Staphylococcus* spp., usually *Staphylococcus intermedius* or *Staphylococcus aureus*.
(c) Therapy involves treatment for 3–6 weeks with an antibiotic which is sensitive to the listed organisms. Recurrence is common, especially if the underlying aetiology has not been detected and treated.

172 (a) The most probable diagnosis is dietary allergy (food hypersensitivity). Other differential diagnoses that should be considered include flea bit allergy, drug hypersensitivity and hypereosinophilic syndrome.
(b) The diagnosis is made by feeding the patient a low allergen diet for a minimum of 6 weeks. Hypoallergenic diets must be individualised for each patient based upon careful dietary history-taking. The objective is to feed the patient foodstuffs which have not previously been fed. The diet should also be free of additives, colourings, flavourings and preservatives. In the cat, palatability is a common problem; rabbit and venison are accepted by some patients.
(c) Food hypersensitivity in the cat may also present as miliary dermatitis, generalised pruritus, urticaria and angioedema, pruritic seborrhoeic skin disease, lesions of the eosinophilic granuloma complex, self-induced alopecia and pruritic otitis externa.

173 (a) The most likely diagnosis is a mycetoma. The triad of swelling, draining fistulas and tissue granules is very suggestive of a mycetoma. Other differential diagnoses to consider would include phaeohyphomycosis, foreign body and tumour.
(b) There are two diagnostic tests required to confirm the diagnosis. The first test is a biopsy to confirm histologically that the lesion is a mycetoma. Classic histological findings include diffuse-to-nodular inflammation with tissue granules. The fungal hyphae comprise the tissue granules. The second test is culture of a section of the tissue on both Sabouraud's dextrose agar and blood agar. Mycetomas may be caused by fungi (eumycotic mycetomas) or by actinomycetes (filamentous bacteria, e.g. *Nocardia*).
(c) If the mycetoma is caused by a bacterial organism, surgical drainage and appropriate antimicrobial therapy may be curative. However, in the case of fungal mycetomas, amputation of the affected area is often the most effective therapy.

174 (a) The most likely diagnosis is allergic contact dermatitis or contact hypersensitivity. If one of the products used on this patient had been a contact 'irritant', other dogs treated in the same fashion would have developed skin problems.
(b) In most cases, contact hypersensitivity represents a type IV (delayed) hypersensitivity reaction.
(c) Therapy of contact hypersensitivity in the dog and cat includes avoidance of the offending allergen. Many times, the allergen is quite difficult to identify. This particular patient should be bathed in a hypoallergenic shampoo. A short course of systemic glucocorticoids would be beneficial in alleviating this patient's discomfort.

175 (a)   The canine scabies mite (*Sarcoptes scabiei* var. *canis*) is capable of burrowing in human skin, laying eggs, depositing faeces and the eggs maturing to the larval stage. It is assumed that the canine scabies mite is not capable of completing its life cycle on human skin. The burrowing, egg-laying and faeces deposition result in intense pruritus for most humans 'infested' with canine scabies.

(b)   The 'naked' mites live for only a few hours in the environment. However, if a large scab is scratched off the host and contains viable mites, these are capable of living in the environment for several days.

(c)   The canine scabies mite has become resistant to numerous insecticides over the years. In the United States, patients infected with the mite are best treated with weekly amitraz dips for 6 weeks, or with subcutaneous Ivermectin (Bovine Ivomec®) every 2 weeks for six treatments. Before treating canine scabies patients, please be aware of the potentially adverse side effects of the above-mentioned drugs.

(d)   If the owner of the scabetic canine is uncomfortable, it is best that he/she seeks the advice of his/her general practitioner. Even though we as veterinarians may have very helpful treatment suggestions, this is not our purpose. 'Helpful hints' may not be helpful, and may be dangerous!

176 (a)   Feline acne, chin acne.

(b)   Idiopathic, allergic, demodicosis, dermatophyte infection, and bacterial infection.

(c)   Complete physical examination is usually diagnostic. However, a definitive diagnosis may be made via skin biopsies submitted for histopathologic examination.

(d)   Topical therapy with 3% benzoyl peroxide shampoo and/or anti-seborrhoeic shampoos (without tar) would be beneficial, but they are quite difficult to apply to the chin of cats and even more difficult to convince the cat to leave them on! Systemic glucocorticoids (subcutaneous methyl prednisone acetate at a dosage of 4 – 5 mg/kg) are quite beneficial, but frequent use may cause very severe side effects. In some cases, systemic antibiotics are beneficial. 'hot-packing' is helpful, but many cats will not allow this. Since the underlying aetiology is very difficult to find, and therefore difficult/impossible to treat, symptomatic therapy may be the best course of action despite its deficiencies.

177 (a)   Pemphigus foliaceus, zinc dermatopathy, bacterial folliculitis and superficial necrolytic dermatosis.

(b)   Zinc dermatopathy ('zinc-responsive' dermatosis).

(c)   Skin biopsies taken for histopathologic examination in 10% buffered formalin are usually diagnostic. The biopsies reveal extensive parakeratosis (retained nuclei in the stratum corneum), with a slightly acanthotic epidermis.

(d)   This patient's diet contains enough zinc for the 'normal' dog. For some reason, this amount is not sufficient for this particular patient. Reasons may include poor absorption of zinc from the intestinal tract, an abnormally high requirement for dietary zinc and food additives (such as calcium), which bind to the zinc and prevent its absorption. There are various zinc supplements available. Some are listed here:

1 Zinc gluconate. 2 Zinc sulphate. 3 Zinc methionate. 4 Zin pro*.

All forms of zinc may cause nausea and are therefore best divided into BID dosages and given with some food. Unfortunately, not all patients diagnosed with a zinc-'responsive' dermatopathy respond to zinc. The reasons for this are not known.

178 (a)   Hepatoid gland adenoma. Other names for this tumour are perianal gland adenoma and circumanal gland adenoma.

(b)   The best treatment is surgical excision. Other forms of therapy that are used are:

1 Cryosurgery (care must be taken to prevent damage to the anal sphincter muscles. Damage to these muscles usually results in permanent faecal incontinence. For most owners, this renders a

dog an 'unacceptable pet'). 2 Intralesional injections of diethylstilbesterol (DES) have been used, but side effects include bone marrow suppression (which may be permanent) and prostatic squamous metaplasia. 3 Radiation therapy is quite useful in cases which are not amendable to surgical excision.

(c) Neutering the dog to remove the primary source of tumour-inciting androgens is extremely important.

179 (a) Dermatophyte infection, pemphigus foliaceus, systemic lupus erythematosus, and drug eruption.

(b) Skin biopsies for histopathologic examination, submitted in 10% buffered formalin, skin biopsies for direct immunofluorescence submitted in Michel's media, and a fungal culture.(The diagnosis was pemphigus foliaceus.)

180 (a) Colour mutant/dilution alopecia, 'blue' Dobermann syndrome. (Also seen in fawn Dobermanns).

(b) Very dull, dry, sparse hair coat, mainly involving the dorsal midline and lateral thoracic areas. These patients frequently have secondary seborrhoeic abnormalities and secondary bacterial folliculitis and furunculosis.

(c) There is no treatment for the 'disease' itself. This abnormal coat is associated with the genes for blue and fawn colour in Dobermann pinschers. Since many Dobermanns are hypothyroid, this should be investigated, as hypothyroidism would exacerbate the clinical signs. Antibiotics are indicated when secondary bacterial infection is present. In some cases of recurrent bacterial infection associated with genetic dilution, staph bacterin injections are helpful.

Note: The editor believes that there really are no normal-coated blue or fawn Dobermanns.

181 (a) These tumours are benign and slow growing. They frequently ulcerate and develop secondary bacterial infection. The tumours may be painful, odiferous and unsightly, but they do not metastasize.

(b) Norwegian elkhound and Keeshond.

182 (a) Is the amount of bruising more extensive than should be expected for the amount of sustained trauma?

(b) If the answer to (a) is yes, then numerous diseases which result in increased clotting time should be considered, such as: hyperadrenocorticism, Von Willebrand's disease, rickettsial diseases and adverse drug reactions.

183 (a) Thermal or chemical burn, pemphigus vulgaris, systemic lupus erythematosus and vasculitis.

(b) Drugs (including vaccines) and internal neoplastic disease.

184 (a) Internal metabolic disease, diabetes mellitus, severe vacuolar hepatopathy, pancreatic tumours and other neoplastic disease.

(b) Treatment of the skin disease must be based upon detecting and treating the underlying internal disease. This is often quite difficult and frustrating, and many of the associated internal diseases are not treatable.

185 (a) Phaeohyphomycosis. This is an uncommon subcutaneous infection caused by dematiaceous (pigmented) septate fungi. This disease differs from mycetomas in that there are no tissue granules.

(b) If the lesion is located on a limb, amputation of the limb is the treatment of choice. If the lesion is not on a part of the patient that cannot be non-lethally amputated, very wide surgical excision is necessary. In some cases, intralesional amphoterocin B, fluorocytosine, ketoconazole, and itraconazole have been somewhat effective. In general, medical management is much more difficult than surgical excision.

(c)   For this patient, the prognosis is guarded. The lesion is not located on a limb that can be amputated. If surgically removed, recurrences at the surgical site are quite common.

186   (a)   Follicular dysplasia/hypotrichosis of the Irish water spaniel.
(b)   Skin biopsies for histopathologic examination.
(c)   None. The alopecia is permanent.

187   (a)   Idiopathic Cocker (American) seborrhoea.
(b)   Diagnosis is based upon the breed of dog, skin biopsies for histopathologic examination and ruling out other possible similar and/or complicating diseases such as hypothyroidism, food hypersensitivity, allergic inhalant disease (atopy) and vitamin A-responsive dermatosis. Skin biopsies reveal severe acanthosis and hyperkeratosis. There is also follicular keratosis and the presence of ostia (openings) of the follicles. Dermal inflammation has both a mononuclear and neutrophilic infiltrate.
(c)   There is no cure for this condition and treatment is usually very frustrating. The abnormal sebaceous secretion predisposes the patient to chronic recurrent bacterial and yeast skin/ear infections. These are treated with systemic antibiotics as well as a systemic anti-fungal medication (ketoconazole at a dosage of 6 – 10 mg/kg once daily for 20 days). Keeping the hair coat clipped short and weekly anti-seborrhoeic baths are very helpful. Corticosteroids have two very beneficial effects: they reduce the abnormal sebaceous secretion and decease the patient's pruritus. Obviously, care must be used in monitoring the side effects of long-term use of the medications required to allow these patients to live a relatively comfortable (but certainly not drug-free) life.
Note: A small number of these patients benefit from systemic retinoid (etretinate) therapy. This drug is quite expensive and must be closely monitored. Most likely, the Cockers that are helped by this drug are not truly 'Cocker seborrhoeics', but vitamin A-responsive dermatosis cases.

188   (a)   Hyperadrenocorticism (Cushing's syndrome).
(b)   In most cases, a chemistry profile reveals an elevated alkaline phosphatase and a complete blood count shows eosinopenia, neutrophilia and lymphopenia. Confirmation is made by ACTH stimulation testing and/or low-dose, high-dose dexamethasone suppression testing. Abdominal sonograms may reveal an adrenal mass.
(c)   If the disease is not caused by an adrenal tumour, Lysodren® (o,p'-DDD) is the treatment of choice. Secondary bacterial skin infection, when present, requires long-term, systemic antibiotic therapy. Some patients develop secondary demodicosis, which requires weekly amitraz dips.
(d)   The Boston terrier, Miniature Poodle, Boxer and Dachshund are at increased risk of developing this disease.

189   (a)   Multiple apocrine cysts.
(b)   Some of these cysts may arise due to blockage of the apocrine duct. However, a significant portion of these cases occur in old dogs and may be a 'senile' change.

190   (a)   Bacterial hypersensitivity, staphylococcal hypersensitivity.
(b)   The probable causative organism is a coagulase-positive *Staphylococcus* spp., usually *Staphylococcus intermedius*. Rarely, a coagulase-negative *Staphylococcus* spp. is isolated.
(c)   Bacterial folliculitis, demodicosis, dermatophytosis, seborrhoeic skin disease, subcorneal pustular dermatosis, sterile eosinophilic pustulosis, pemphigus foliaceus, systemic lupus erythematosus, allergic inhalant disease (atopy), food hypersensitivity, sarcoptic mange and flea bite hypersensitivity.

191 (a) Flea collar contact dermatitis.

(b) Treatment involves removing the offending collar and clipping the hair from the affected areas. Wet dressings may be used if the lesions are severe. Usually systemic, short-acting cortisone is necessary for several days to decrease inflammation and pruritus. In mild cases, topical cortisone may be sufficient. Protecting the area from self-trauma with a loose stockinet is helpful. If the area is secondarily infected, systemic antibiotics are indicated.

(c) Several steps may be taken to prevent this condition. These include: 1 Removing the flea collar from the airtight package and allowing it to 'air out' for 24 – 48 hours before placing it on the pet. 2 The collar should be placed loosely around the neck, allowing four fingers to be easily slid under the collar. 3 Other flea control methods may be used. The flea collar is really helpful in preventing flea bites in cats and dogs under 8 kg of body weight. The collar is quite helpful in preventing the attachment of ticks around the neck and ears of any sized dog or cat. (If the patient is flea-allergic and weighs over 8 kg, the flea collar should not be used.)

192 (a) Benign. These tumours rarely recur at the site of surgical excision. There have been very rare reports of metastasis (possible misdiagnosis?).

(b) Digits, ears, lips and mucocutaneous junctions.

193 (a) Sporotrichosis. Any cat with an exudative, non-healing wound should be evaluated for possible infection with *Sporotrix schenckii*. The organism may or may not be present in large numbers in the exudate. Culture and cytologic examination should always be performed.

(b) The treatment of choice is sodium iodide. However, cats are very sensitive to iodides and therapy must be carefully monitored. In humans, itraconazole is usually effective.

(c) The owner must be warned that this is a serious zoonotic disease.

194 Pemphigus foliaceus, cutaneous lymphosarcoma, nutritional deficiencies, intestinal parasites, too frequent bathing, dermatophyte infection and a myriad of internal diseases with cutaneous signs.

195 (a) Skin scrapings for mites.

(b) The mite *Demodex canis*.

(c) Weekly amitraz dippings until the mites are eliminated. This may require from 6 to greater than 30 weekly dippings, depending upon the severity of the disease in the particular patient.

(d) Localised demodicosis, which is defined as five or less areas of the body that are skin scraping positive for demodex canis, is not hereditary. It is usually related to 'stress', such as sex hormone changes, boarding, dog show circuits etc. Generalised demodicosis, as defined by the American Academy of Veterinary Dermatology, is positive skin scrapings involving greater than five body areas. This form of the disease is considered to be hereditary, and affected dogs (male and female) should not be used in breeding programmes.

196 (a) Intracutaneous cornifying epithelioma and epidermal inclusion cyst.

(b) Keratin.

(c) Wide surgical excision is the treatment of choice if the lesions are few in number. If large numbers of masses are found on the patient, isotretinoin (1.7 – 4 mg/kg/day) and etretinate (1.1 – 1.5 mg/kg/day) have been found to be helpful in some patients with intracutaneous cornifying epithelioma.

(d) Rupture of the tumour or cyst, with release of the keratinous material into the surrounding dermis, evokes a marked pyogranulomatous inflammatory response.

(e) The Norwegian elkhound.

197 (a) Erythema multiforme and toxic epidermal necrolysis secondary to injectable gold salt therapy.

(b) Multiple skin biopsies submitted for histopathologic examination in 10% buffered formalin. The histopathologic diagnosis is erythema multiforme, most likely secondary to an adverse drug reaction to the gold salt therapy.

(c) Corticosteroids and/or chlorambucil. (The editor has seen numerous fatal adverse reactions to azathioprine in cats who are correctly dosed and appropriately monitored.)

198 (a) Benign.

(b) Usually multiple.

(c) They may be unsightly, and may be irritated by combing and clipping of the patient.

199 (a) Thermal burn due to a hot water pipe that the patient leaned against in the bathtub, while being bathed.

(b) Scarring at the site of trauma.

200 (a) This lesion is described as a 'target' or 'bull's eye' lesion. The lesion is an annular area of central erythema and/or hyperpigmentation with alopecia and scaling that spreads peripherally. Lesions may coalesce.

(b) Early lesions are erythematous pustules and haemorrhagic bullae.

(c) The pathomechanism of bacterial hypersensitivity in dogs is unclear, although evidence supports the existence of a type III, and perhaps a type I, hypersensitivity reaction

201 (a) Fibrosarcoma.

(b) Many feline fibrosarcomas are found arising at the sites of intradermal vaccination. The pathomechanism of the development of these tumours is under investigation, but is probably associated with persistence of the antigen and the adjuvant (usually aluminium hydroxide) at the vaccination site.

Editor's note: The recognition of these vaccination-induced tumours is in no way a reason not to vaccinate any feline patient appropriately. The chance of developing a viral disease because of non-vaccination is far greater than the chance of the feline patient developing a fibrosarcoma. Also, rabies is on the rise in many areas of the world, and failure to vaccinate feline patients could result in a zoonotic disaster.

202 (a) Yes. Various intestinal parasites (including ascarids, coccidia, hookworms, tapeworms and whipworms) of dogs, cats and humans have been reported to be associated with pruritic dermatosis.

(b) Diagnosis of intestinal parasite hypersensitivity is made based upon history, physical examination, faecal flotation and response to therapy. Response to therapy is especially important.

(c) Clinical presentations reported in the dog to be associated with intestinal parasite hypersensitivity include:

1 Generalised or multifocal pruritic papulo-crustous dermatitis. 2 Pruritic seborrhoeic skin disease. 3 Pruritic urticaria. 4 Pruritus, without obvious skin lesions.

203 (a) *Blastomyces dermatitides.*

(b) This is a dimorphic fungus that causes systemic infections in animals and humans. A careful ocular examination, as well as radiographs of the chest and abdomen, are the minimal requirements to assess the degree of dissemination of the infection.

(c) No. Blastomycosis is not a zoonotic disease. In cases in which the dogs and owners are infected, a common source of exposure is present.

204 (a) Cutaneous histiocytosis. This is a pseudoneoplastic, histiocytic, proliferative disease of dogs.

(b) The Shetland sheepdog and the collie appear to be at increased risk for developing the disease.

205 (a) Very rare.
(b) At birth.
(c) Males are definitely predisposed.
(d) The Poodle, Beagle, Labrador retriever and Bichon Frise appear to be at increased risk.

206 (a) Telogen defluxion, telogen effluvium.
(b) The history and clinical signs are quite important; however, a definitive diagnosis may be made based only upon skin biopsies submitted in 10% buffered formalin for histopathologic examination.
(c) No treatment is indicated or needed.
(d) Yes. The hair loss is never permanent. Evidence of hair re-growth is usually noticed in 4 – 10 weeks.

207 (a) Skin biopsies submitted for histopathologic examination in 10% buffered formalin are the most important. Second is a blood (serum) test for antinuclear antibody (ANA) levels. Third are skin biopsies submitted in Michel's media for direct immunofluorescence testing. However, the footpads and noses of most normal cats and dogs show positive fluorescence.
(b) Systemic lupus erythematosus.
(c) Glomerulonephritis, lymphadenopathy, fever of unknown origin, weight loss and haemolytic anaemia.

208 (a) Mast cell tumour. This tumour has recurred at the surgical site, which is a common finding in canine mast cell tumours. Note that there are numerous subcutaneous nodules in the hock area, due to tumour extension along lymphatic vessels.
(b) Amputation of the limb.
(c) Metastases are frequently found in the 'draining' lymph nodes. Tumour cells can often be identified in the lymph nodes upon cytologic examination of the node aspirate. The spleen and the liver are the most common sites of distant metastases.

209 (a) Trichoepithelioma and pilomatrixoma.
(b) Both of these tumours show proliferation of primitive germinal cells with differentiation to hair follicular epithelium and 'ghost cells' or 'shadow cells'. Pilomatrixomas, on histopathology, show only central aggregation of 'ghost cells' and multinucleated giant cells. Trichoepitheliomas reveal greater differentiation to more mature hair follicular structures, such as external and internal root sheath epithelium. On histopathology, the tumour shown was a pilomatrixoma.

210 (a) Pemphigus foliaceus.
(b) Skin biopsies submitted for histopathologic examination in 10% buffered formalin are the most important. Skin biopsies in Michel's media for direct immunofluorescence are also important, but many laboratories are not capable of accurately interpreting this test. Also, there are numerous false positives and false negatives.
(c) Prednisolone, at a dosage of 1 mg/kg of body weight twice daily, combined with azathiprine at a dosage of 1 mg/kg once daily, is the treatment of choice. If, after several weeks, this therapy is not effective, the diagnosis should be re-evaluated and if still consistent with pemphigus foliaceous, injectable gold salt therapy should be initiated.

211 (a) Canine follicular dysplasia of the English bulldog or idiopathic flank alopecia.
(b) Skin biopsies for histopathologic examination.
(c) No treatment is helpful.
(d) The Boxer, miniature Schnauzer, Airedale terrier and Dobermann pinscher.

212 (a) Pemphigus erythematosus, pemphigus foliaceus and discoid lupus erythematosus.
(b) Biopsies for histopathologic examination, biopsies for direct immunofluorescence testing and a serum sample for antinuclear antibody testing.
(c) Pemphigus erythematosus.
Comments: PE is an uncommon benign variant of pemphigus foliaceus. There may be some components of systemic lupus erythematosus, since some patients have a positive antinuclear antibody test. This disease has been reported in the dog and cat.

213 (a) Injection reaction alopecia.
(b) Skin biopsies for histopathologic examination will give a definitive diagnosis. However, in most cases, the history of receiving a vaccination (or any injection) within 3 months prior to the onset of the alopecia is usually diagnostic.
(c) In most cases the alopecia is permanent. However, if the owner is concerned about the cosmetic appearance of the 'lesion', it may easily be removed under local anaesthesia in most patients.

214 (a) Abnormal sex hormone (oestrogen) secretion due to retained testes.
(b) Gathering more information from the previous owner (if possible) would obviously be beneficial. Serum sex hormone levels may help to support a diagnosis of 'sex hormone imbalance'. In many cases, exploratory surgery is necessary to look for, and remove, retained testes.

215 (a) Food allergy, allergic inhalant disease (atopy), hypothyroidism, autoimmune disease (such as lupus erythematosus and pemphigus), structural defects such as heavy ear pinnae or stenotic canals (seen in flop-eared dogs, Shar peis and American Cocker spaniels), and flea bite hypersensitivity.
(b) The only way to treat the otitis appropriately is to determine and treat the underlying aetiology(ies). Symptomatic treatment of otitis externa, ignoring the aetiology, is very unrewarding to the veterinarian, owner and patient.

216 (a) Autoimmune skin disease and contact irritant/allergic dermatitis.
(b) It is best to treat the underlying cause. However, scrotal ulcerations are very difficult to heal, and 90% of these patients require neutering with scrotal ablation.

217 (a) The organisms are the larval forms of diphtherous flies. The flies are well known to deposit their eggs on ulcerated, macerated, wet skin. The disease is called myiasis or maggot infestation.
(b) The areas should be clipped gently and cleaned with warm water. Antibiotics are often necessary due to secondary bacterial skin infection (especially in a demodicosis patient).
(c) The patient should be kept inside most of the day. If this is not possible, the area around the patient's pen should be treated on a regular basis with a fly-killing insecticide. There are numerous topical fly-repellents, although these may be contra-indicated in this patient due to the severity of skin ulceration as well as the patient's debilitation.

218 (a) Puppy strangles, puppy cellulitis, juvenile pyoderma.
(b) This disease is believed to be an immune-mediated/ autoimmune skin disease. The editor has seen many dogs develop the disease post-vaccinal. This reaction may be because the patient's immune system is immature and is incapable of reacting/acting appropriately to the injected virus(es) and instead produces self-antibodies.
Note: In no way is this disease a reason for not vaccinating puppies according to accepted vaccination schedules.
(c) The disease is best treated with high dosages of glucocorticoids; 1 – 2 mg per kg of body

weight twice daily for 7 – 10 days, then tapering the dosage over a 6 – 10 week period.

219 (a) This cat is developing cutaneous haemorrhage secondary to bone marrow suppression and resultant thrombocytopenia, secondary to the gold salt therapy. This is a possible, but quite uncommon, adverse reaction to gold salt therapy in the feline.
(b) Obviously, the gold salt therapy should be at least temporarily discontinued. However, the anaemia and thrombocytopenia may continue to progress because the gold salts remain in the body for at least 6 weeks. Therefore, the patient should be evaluated with a complete blood count every 5 – 7 days. Many feline patients do eventually require blood transfusions.
Note: Once the side effects of the gold salts have been treated, the gold salt therapy may be resumed at a lower dosage and increased injection interval. However, the patient must be closely monitored for a recurrence of an adverse reaction.

220 (c).

221 (a).

222 (a) The signalment and clinical signs are highly suggestive of this disorder. The Siberian husky is definitely predisposed. The lesions occur on the lateral or ventral surface of the tongue. The owners often complain of severe, malodorous breath (which is often quite evident). Definitive diagnosis is made by biopsies submitted in 10% buffered formalin for histopathologic examination. Characteristic histopathologic changes include variable size foci of collagen degeneration, eosinophilic and histiocytic cellular infiltration, and palisading granulomas.
(b) Numerous granulomatous and neoplastic disorders.
(c) Canine oral eosinophilic granulomas are usually very glucocorticoid-responsive. 78% of cases treated with prednisone at a dosage of 0.5 – 2.2 mg/kg per day orally showed regression of the lesions within 10 – 20 days. In these cases, no further therapy was needed. In some cases, the lesions regress spontaneously.

223 Unfortunately, the Chinese Shar pei is predisposed to all of the listed skin disorders.

224 (b) Is not true. Present-day antihistamines bind to either the H1 or H2 receptors, but not to both. (c), (d), and (e) are true of antihistamines used in other species, but may or may not have similar clinical applications in the canine patient.

225 All of the listed substances have been reported to cause allergic contact dermatitis in dogs and cats.

226 1 Bacterial skin infection. 2 Seborrhoeic abnormalities. 3 Demodicosis. 4 Calcinosis cutis. 5 Dermatophyte infection.

227 1 Canine cutaneous histiocytoma. 2 Mast cell tumour. 3 Cutaneous lymphosarcoma. 4 Cutaneous plasmacytoma. 5 Transmissible venereal tumour (metastasis to the skin).

228 (a) Unsaturated fatty acids are necessary for caloric energy and the formation and maintenance of the fluidity and the function of cell membranes.
(b) The oxidative metabolism of certain fatty acids results in the formation of eicosanoids, which include the prostaglandins and leucotrienes.
(c) Eicosapentanoic acid (EPA), found in marine lipids, is metabolized to the three-series of eicosanoids which is believed to be anti-inflammatory.
(d) Linoleic, arachadonic and linolenic acids are essential fatty acids. The dog can synthesise both arachadonic and linolenic acids from linoleic acid.
(e) In general, reports using fatty acids as therapy in canines with allergic inhalant disease (atopy) have shown a decrease in clinical signs and improvement of the hair coat, but certainly

not (in most cases) the cessation of pruritus.

229 (e) Basset hound. (a) Siberian husky. (f) Kerry Blue terrier. (b) giant Schnauzer. (c) Norwegian elkhound. (d) American Cocker spaniel.

230 (c) Calcinosis cutis.

231 (a) The tail (both the dorsal and ventral surfaces) is a common site.
(b) The ventral abdomen, primarily in the periprepucial areas.
(c) The hind limbs.
(d) The back or dorsal midline.
Note: Very occasionally, these tumours may occur on the head and neck. Because of their potential widespread distribution on the body, the term 'perianal gland tumour' is also referred to as hepatoid gland tumour.

232 (a) Over 90% of the reported cases of hormonal hypersensitivity (which is an uncommon-to-rare canine disorder) have occurred in intact female dogs.
(b) It is believed that type I and type IV hypersensitivity reactions to endogenous progesterone, oestrogen and/or testosterone are involved.
(c) Therapy includes ovariohysterectomy or neutering. Treatment of secondary seborrhoeic and/or bacterial/yeast dermatologic problems is essential.

233 (a) Meibomian gland adenoma.
(b) Meibomian or tarsal gland.
(c) Sebaceous gland.

234 1 Gastrointestinal ulceration. This may occur as a result of histaminaemia, due to massive release of histamine from the neoplastic mast cells. The histaminaemia increases gastric acid production, damages the endothelium of the gastric vessels which causes intravascular thrombi, producing ischemic necrosis and gastric ulcer development.
2 Local haemorrhage at the site of cutaneous mast cell removal due to heparin release from the neoplastic mast cells.
3 Delayed wound healing at the site of cutaneous mast cell removal due to release of factors that retard fibroplasia.
4 Shock, due to massive and rapid degranulation of mast cells, from either excessive manipulation of the tumour at the time of surgery, or the use of chemotherapeutic agents that cause necrosis of the tumour tissue.

235 (a) Rhodesian Ridgeback.
(b) Simple recessive.
(c) Young dogs, usually less than 18 months of age.
(d) Dorsal midline.
(e) Dermoid sinuses are developmental abnormalities of the neural tube, resulting in incomplete separation of the neural tube and skin during embryonic development.

236 (a) Short wave ultraviolet light (UVB) is the most likely aetiology of squamous cell carcinomas in man and animals.
(b) Chronic sun exposure is a prerequisite for the development of these tumours. In addition, lack of skin pigment, sparse hair or lack of hair allows the ultraviolet rays to penetrate the epidermis and damage the DNA of keratinocytes.
(c1) Ear pinnae, eyelid and planum nasale.
(c2) Ventral abdomen and scrotum.

237 (e) Boxer. (d) Scottish terrier. (f) American Cocker spaniel. (a) Shetland sheepdog. (c)

German shepherd dog. (b) Airedale terrier.

238 (a) Bite hypersensitivity.
(b) Anal sacculitis.
(c) Irritating shampoos, insecticides and chemicals.
(d) Allergic inhalant disease (atopy).
(e) Poor grooming, especially matted hair.
(f) Otitis externa.
(g) Food hypersensitivity.
(h) Intestinal parasite hypersensitivity.
(i) Arthritis or other joint pain.
(j) Foreign bodies.

239 (a) Schnauzer comedo syndrome.
(b) The clinical appearance of the lesions, as well as the breed predisposition, is quite helpful. However, a definitive diagnosis can be made only via skin biopsies submitted for histopathologic examination. The biopsies reveal diffuse distension of the hair follicle with keratin. Secondary folliculitis and furunculosis (usually bacterial) may also be found.
(c) These cases are not curable, only treatable. Routine bathing with follicular flushing shampoos that contain benzoyl peroxide is most helpful. These patients will occasionally require a course of systemic antibiotics to treat secondary bacterial folliculitis. Keeping the hair coat clipped short, especially over the mid-back, is helpful.

240 (a) This cutaneous feline reaction is miliary dermatitis.
(b) There are several causes of miliary dermatitis in the cat. These include: flea bite hypersensitivity, allergic inhalant disease (atopy), food hypersensitivity, drug hypersensitivity, intestinal parasite hypersensitivity, feline hypereosinophilic syndrome, ectoparasite infestation (cheyletiellosis, otodectic mange, trombiculidiasis, cat fur mite, pediculosis), dermatophyte infections (ringworm), staphylococcal infections and dietary imbalances. Flea allergy dermatitis is the most common cause of this reaction pattern in the feline.
(c) The diagnosis of flea allergy dermatitis in the cat is best made by finding fleas and flea excreta on the patient using a flea comb, as well as by positive reaction to intradermally injected flea saliva antigen. Beneficial response to flea control is also a very useful diagnostic aid. Since the cat is often such a meticulous groomer, finding fleas and flea excreta may be impossible; therefore, response to flea control is quite beneficial.

241 (a) The two major differential diagnoses are adult-onset hyposomatotropism (growth hormone-responsive alopecia) and hypo-oestrogenism (oestrogen-responsive alopecia, ovarian imbalance type II).
(b) Since it is almost impossible to have serum testing for growth hormone 'deficiency', a trial course of oestrogen therapy would be helpful in differentiating between the two diagnoses.
(c) Administration of oral diethyl stilbesterol at a dosage of 0.2 mg per 10 kg of body weight once daily for 2 weeks, every other day for 2 weeks, then twice weekly for an additional 8 weeks. (If the patient is oestrogen-responsive, hair re-growth should be noticed starting at 8 – 12 weeks.) If the patient is responsive, in order to maintain the hair coat the oestrogen needs to be administered usually at a dosage of 0.2 mg per 10 kg of body weight every 7 – 14 days.
(d) A complete blood count, including a platelet count, should be taken initially every month for the first 4 months, then every 3 – 6 months. Oestrogen therapy may cause bone marrow suppression in some dogs. Also, some patients will show signs of stress. Since this is only a cosmetic skin disease and has no other associated medical problems, the owner should be well informed of the pros and cons of therapy.

242 (a) Idiopathic flank alopecia. This is one of the many follicular dysplasias which include several alopecic skin diseases, which clinically resemble endocrine imbalances. Many breeds may be affected, but Boxers, English bulldogs, Airedale terriers and miniature Schnauzers appear to be predisposed.

(b) Diagnosis is made on the basis of the patient having a history of a cyclical pattern of waxing and waning alopecia involving the flanks, as well as ruling out endocrine imbalances and performing skin biopsies for histopathologic examination.

(c) No therapy is effective, nor is one really needed, as this skin condition causes patients neither discomfort nor any internal disease. (If the patient is a show dog, this condition can be a devastating one.)

243 (a) Drug eruption, most likely toxic epidermal necrolysis (ten), secondary to the administration of cephalosporin antibiotics.

(b) Drugs responsible for causing adverse cutaneous reactions may be administered orally, topically, by injection or by inhalation. (Most patients have a reaction to orally administered drugs, simply because this is the most common route of administration in the canine and feline.)

(c) Skin biopsies submitted for histopathologic examination would reveal the microscopic changes characteristic of an adverse drug reaction. Unfortunately, the biopsies are not capable of identifying the aetiologic agent.

(d) The treatment consists of immediately withdrawing the suspected drug. Corticosteroids appear to be beneficial in some patients. Supportive care such as cleansing the lesions, providing whirlpool baths and encouraging the patient to eat and drink is important. Unfortunately, almost 50% of patients with drug-induced toxic epidermal necrolysis die.

244 (a) Gynaecomastia, pendulous prepuce, decreased interest in mating, bilaterally symmetric truncal alopecia, attraction of other male dogs to the patient and varying degrees of hyperpigmentation.

(b) Palpation of the testes. At least 50% of these patients have either palpable testicular tumours or abnormalities in the size and/or consistency of the testes.

(c) Even though approximately 50% of patients have palpably normal testes, the apparent cause is abnormal oestrogen secretion by the testes, often by Sertoli-cell tumours.

245 (a) Sebaceous hyperplasia. On histopathology, the cross-section of the lesion revealed an area of inflammation at the base of the hyperplastic sebaceous glands. This is due to the rupture of one of the ducts which convey the secretory material from the glands to the epidermal surface. The secretory material and the keratin from the sebaceous duct evoke a pyogranulomatous inflammatory patient response.

(b) Sebaceous hyperplasia is considered to be a 'senile' change. The lesions do not become cancerous nor metastasize. The most common owner complaints are that the lesions are unsightly and/or are injured and ulcerated during routine grooming procedures. Removal of these lesions can be performed easily under local anaesthesia if the owner wishes. However, the owner should be informed that it is highly likely that new sebaceous hyperplasias will develop as the patient ages.

246 (a) Skin scrapings are the diagnostic test of choice. However, in at least 40% of scabetic canines the mites, eggs or faeces cannot be found despite numerous skin scrapings. The reasons for negative skin scrapings include dislodging of the mites from their epidermal burrows via intense scratching and the fact that low numbers of mites may cause intense pruritus and severe clinical signs in a hypersensitive patient. Response to therapy is often a confirmative diagnostic test.

(b) The kennel should be quarantined until the infestation is eliminated. The premises should be thoroughly sprayed with an insecticide that is formulated to kill fleas. (It is thought that the scabies mite is incapable of living in the environment for more than a few hours. However, the mites are capable of living in large scabs and crusts that have been scratched off the patient for many days, even weeks.) All dogs should be treated for at least 6 – 8 weeks with an 'appropriate' scabicide. Treatments include ivermectin, malathion or amitraz. It is very important to be aware of the fact that there are regional differences in the susceptibility of the mite to various insecticides. (Also, breed sensitivities to certain drugs certainly exist. Ivermectin should not be used for collies, Shetland sheepdogs and possibly other breeds of dogs.)

247 (a) Sertoli-cell tumour of one or both of the retained testicles. (Actually, the assumption by the new owner and veterinarian that the dog had been surgically neutered was incorrect.)
(b) An abdominal mass may be found radiographically or with ultrasound. In some cases, but certainly not all, the patient has elevated serum oestrogen levels.
(c) After a thorough physical examination, complete blood count and chemistry profile, exploratory surgery of the abdomen to look for and remove the retained testicles is recommended.
Note: Retained testicles (or testicle) is considered in most breeds of dogs to be a hereditary condition. Obviously, if the patient has one scrotal testicle, he should not be used for breeding.

248 (a) The alopecic areas have numerous very fine stubbly hairs. Some of these hairs may be plucked out and placed on a glass slide with mineral oil and examined under the microscope. If the alopecia is self-induced, the hairs will have normal hair bulbs and frayed ends.
(b) Flea bite allergy, food allergy and allergic inhalant disease (atopy).
(c) Feline endocrine alopecia. Note: feline endocrine alopecia is extremely rare. Less than 1% of cats presenting with hair loss have endocrine disorders.

249 (a) Generic dog food dermatosis.
(b) Confirmation of the diagnosis may be made by one of two means: by changing the dog food to a well-balanced one or by submitting skin biopsies for histopathologic examination in 10% buffered formalin. Histopathology reveals varying degrees of parakeratosis (retained nuclei in the stratum corneum), dyskeratosis (epidermal cells keratinising at an accelerated rate from that of the surrounding cells) and necrolysis of the superficial epidermis.
(c) No specific therapy is necessary other than changing the diet. Obvious improvement in skin lesions should be noted within 2 – 4 weeks of dietary change.

250 (a) Lipomas.
(b) The tumours are benign. They may be of cosmetic significance in short-coated dogs. Surgical removal is not recommended unless the tumour impedes locomotion (i.e. axillary area) or grows so large that it causes 'imbalance' (i.e. a 4.5 kg tumour on the right thoracic area of a 13.6 kg dog). Female dogs are predisposed to the development of these tumours, which are multiple in about 10% of canine patients.

INDEX
Numbers refer to question and answer numbers.